What People Are Saying About
Chandra Ziegler and *Extraordinary Endurance*

"A short stroll through Chandra's writing reveals that she's a kindred spirit—with creation, Creator, and all who long for harmony. She simultaneously elicits both awe and inspiration, and we are all better for having pondered with her."

— Amanda Rasner, Fortune Lake Lutheran Camp Director

"Reading *Extraordinary Endurance* felt as though a wise and dear friend was holding my hand, guiding, and comforting me as I reclaimed my balance. In 2020, I felt like the world was spinning out of control and finding balance was challenging. We all need role models who can coach us on 'getting the most out of every day.' Ms. Ziegler offers knowledge, support, and passion on how to find personal balance and how to plant seeds of peace, joy, and love in the world. I will return to *Extraordinary Endurance*'s personal stories, quotations, poetry, and training tips frequently to sustain my own sense of balance."

— N. Suzanne Standerford, PhD, Distinguished Professor Emeritus, Northern Michigan University, School of Education

"With the chakras as scaffolding, Chandra takes you on a journey into yourself through her story. This joyfully illustrated book feels like a warm hug, and if you journal along with her brilliant prompts, you'll emerge with your own extraordinary endurance, ready to blossom no matter what."

— Sarah Bamford Seidelmann, MD, Author of *Swimming with Elephants: My Unexpected Pilgrimage from Physician to Healer*

"Chandra's weaving of personal narrative, poetry, and resources, combined with the elegant illustrations is like an elixir for my weary soul. As a fellow educator and athlete with a spiritual and creative heart, this book hit close to home on so many levels. The words and images give us gifts of honesty and wisdom. *Extraordinary Endurance* is like a box filled with treasures and reminders and *hope* that I will return to again and again."

— Melissa Hronkin, Former National Elementary Art Educator of the Year

"Chandra Ziegler's *Extraordinary Endurance* is that rare mix of inspiration, wisdom, and practical life experience that will make you feel you have met someone who understands the craziness of life, but more importantly, has learned to handle it with grace. From skiing and running marathons to being a teacher and raising a family, Chandra shares the moments that bring joy and teach resilience. This book will show you how to relax, enjoy the ride, and celebrate life once again!"

— Tyler R. Tichelaar, PhD and award-winning author of *Spirit of the North* and *When Teddy Came to Town*

Extraordinary Endurance

A Training Plan for the Marathon of Life

You are extraordinary

By Chandra Ziegler

Illustrations by Melanie Bess-Haight

Extraordinary Endurance:
A Training Plan for the Marathon of Life

Published by: Dream Star Dragonfly

Address all inquiries to:
Chandra Ziegler
chandraziegler@gmail.com
www.DreamStarDragonfly.com

ISBN: 978-0-578-87833-1

Editors: Tyler Tichelaar and Larry Alexander,
Superior Book Productions

Cover Design: Melanie Bess-Haight

Interior Book Layout: Larry Alexander, Superior Book Productions

Every attempt has been made to source properly all quotes.

Dedication

To the most extraordinary loves of my life,
Erich, Emma, Hali, and Kate.

This book is for anyone who wants to bring more joy into their lives, who wants to live life with total authenticity and beauty and get the most out of every waking moment, who has a dream (or two or twenty) in their heart but needs that little nudge to go after it, who doesn't have a dream or forgot how to dream, who just needs a little hope while enduring all that life has thrown their way. This book is for endurance athletes and non-endurance athletes alike. This book is for you!

So, get comfortable with it. Go on a picture walk. (Sorry, that's my elementary teacher voice speaking.) Soak in all the positive vibes because, Lord knows, I poured a *lot* of energy into these pages you're holding, and we need all the positivity we can get.

My hope and prayer is that the stories and messages in this book will help propel you into living your best life. I want you to live your happiest life and achieve all your dreams. You know why? Because when each of us collectively is full of positive energy, we can change the world!

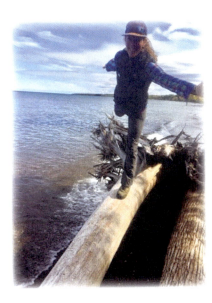

Love,
Chandra

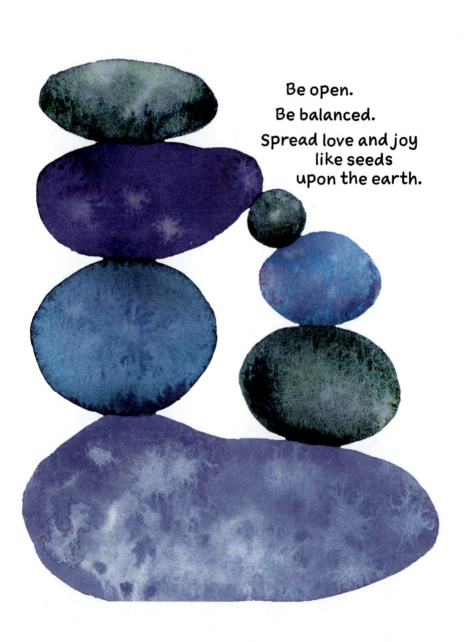

Be open.
Be balanced.
Spread love and joy
like seeds
upon the earth.

Introduction

How many of you have ever participated in a marathon? Okay. How many of you have ever run a 5K? All right, now be honest here; how many of you have ever run either without a training plan? If so, how successful were you? If you haven't run either, can you imagine how successful others were without a training plan?

I'm sure a few people have signed up for an event on a whim, and then when race day rolled around, they were like, "Well, shit, I paid for this; I didn't have time to train, but I might as well do it." So they finished. Woohoo. But how well do you think they really did? Do you think they could've done better?

Absofuckenlutely

Had our hypothetical person had a plan and stuck with it, they would have done a hundred times better! I'm not saying everything should be planned out, and I'm not saying every race needs to be run to set a PR (personal record), but having a few guideposts to help you on your journey makes life a little more manageable, enjoyable, and purposeful. As a society, we frankly need to live more *inspired*!

I've done thirty marathons: two mountain biking, four running, two trail running, the rest skiing. My goal is to do fifty by the time I'm fifty.... I'm currently thirty-six years old. I'm getting there! I did ski marathons without a plan because I like to enjoy myself (and give myself some grace when I'm not able to ski super-long distances in the winter), and frankly, because you can glide once in a while and rest.

Don't get me wrong. I'm super-competitive, and I want to do my best. I love skiing. One of these days, I'll commit to training for a ski marathon and see just how well I can do. Running, on the other hand, is trickier. I know I can't fudge my way through 26.2 miles. Trust me…I tried once…not by choice…but by sheer grit and stubborn determination to finish what I had started. I've followed many, many plans, and I know what it takes to reach whatever goal I set.

To you, that may sound painfully boring or just plain painful. Or maybe not. I don't judge. If you're an endurance sport fanatic like myself…high-five! If not, that's cool too. I have friends from all walks of life, and I would like to count you as my friend too. Whatever the case may be, having a plan helps.

But this book is not just about running a race; it's about living life with your best foot forward and getting the most out of every day. Which is why the subtitle of this book is "A Training Plan for the Marathon of Life."

This book is organized into seven sections, each linked to a specific chakra. Basically, the seven main chakras are specific points along your spine from your sit bone up to the crown of your head. Each is connected to specific organs in your body, as well as different physical, physiological, emotional, and spiritual states of being. The chakras are a spiritual energy center, and they have been referenced and used for thousands of years.

Each section of this book plays an important role in your overall training plan.

I begin with blank space and invite you to pause and simply breathe. To ground and center yourself. To let go of all the thoughts spinning in your mind and just be present. You need to show up for yourself at a very deep level to make this training plan work. Only *you* can do the work.

Then I share a brief visualization for you to repeat silently in your mind. This is a great way to begin a meditation session.

I go on to share some stories from my life. Perhaps they'll show you in a real way how to apply that specific training tip, or they'll show you how I failed and kept trying anyway.

I continue each section with a quote and some guiding questions to get you thinking about that particular chakra and how it relates to your body, mind, and spirit, your relationships with other people and God, and your place in the world.

After the exercise, I provide training tips for each chakra to encourage you to act. I provide a list of energizing and healing activities for you to choose from to help bring about the desired change you seek. The training tips will support you physically, emotionally, and spiritually. They will raise your vibration, and you will begin to live at a higher frequency. You'll begin to tune in to your true desires and live more intentionally. Basically, you'll begin to feel like a million bucks…or at least be smiling a bit more.

What training tips are included?

Visualizations: Words to read to help you visualize and grow

Affirmations: Words to repeat to help you stay grounded

Crystal Therapy: Crystals to wear or carry to add to your natural healing toolkit

Nutrition: Foods to eat to benefit your physical body

Aromatherapy: Essential oils to diffuse or inhale to support all systems

Sound Therapy: Things to listen to that promote healing

Yoga Poses: Asanas to hold to encourage flexibility and strength

Healing with Nature: Ways to connect with our Mother Earth

For more details about any of these training tips, I provide further information in the resource section at the back of the book. All the suggestions are extremely valuable and have healing power, but you need to do what feels right for you in whichever season of life you're in. Amen? A successful training plan allows the *trainee*…you…some choice and flexibility. If one of the ideas speaks more to you than others, by all means, do it every day. Come back to these whenever you're feeling stuck or need a boost of energy.

Next, I encourage you to use the blank "Be Extraordinary" pages to draw, take notes, ask questions, and keep track of the shifts you experience, miracles you witness, and signs from all around you - anything that inspires you to live your best life.

Finally, keep your high vibe going and practice some mindfulness while you color a beautiful creation from my amazing illustrator, Melanie.

I encourage you to doodle all over the book, write in the margins, and highlight. If it feels good, do it.

Maybe on your butterfly-like journey of transformation you're in the egg stage. You might be happy where you are, in your cozy surroundings, so you don't want anything to change—or you might be feeling trapped and can't wait to get out. Or perhaps you're at the caterpillar stage. You have left your comfort zone and taken a step in faith into a bigger world of possibilities, but you find yourself crawling through life—still with purpose, but crawling, nonetheless.

Never doubt that powerful forces are at play and change is always happening. You will begin to feel yourself going through a powerful metamorphosis. In the chrysalis stage, you might revert to the state of mind you had when you were just an egg. You might begin to let fear hold you back. You must simply embrace the darkness, knowing what fabulous illumination lies ahead.

Soon enough, you'll feel yourself begin to crack out of that cocoon and emerge as an exquisite butterfly, ready to fly. But even at this stage, there is still work to be done. Wherever you are is where you're meant to be in the circle of life. Just begin. I believe with my whole heart that this book will help guide you on your journey of transformation.

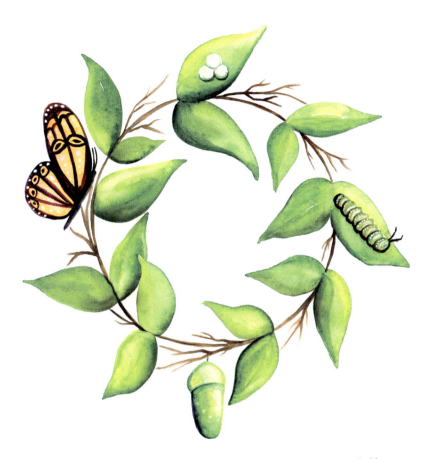

Ultimately, everyone is different and will react in different ways to the same thing. I encourage you to take the path of least resistance when it comes to dealing with any issue. Heal yourself by using what you already have…a body, a mind, and a spirit. Incorporate natural modes of healing, which I recommend in each section. Jump ahead if you wish, or keep reading sequentially. It's up to you. It's *always* up to you! Remember, you're training for life here…so take your time. Come back to this training plan at any point and reread any section you need to attend to a little more earnestly.

If you're reading about chakras or alternative methods of healing for the first time, I suggest you start with your root chakra. Read the chapter, sit and meditate on the topic, do the journal entries, try the yoga poses, and see what you think.

Notice how you feel. Take the time to focus on grounding yourself for about a week before you move on to the next chakra. If you feel ready after a few days, by all means, read on.

If you want to skip right to the activities to help with an issue you're having, please do. However, perhaps it makes more sense for you to read the whole thing first—to see how everything fits together and is connected. Just know you will do no harm by going out of order.

During times of complete upheaval, uncertainty, stress, and change, I often meditate on the chakras. Doing so provides a sort of tangible focus for my highly charged emotional self. I'll sit in the quiet of the morning and start with my root chakra and slowly scan my whole body. I visualize the place in my body, the beautiful color related to that region, and ask myself specific chakra-related questions, such as: How will you stay grounded today? How will you soak up the beauty and joy of the present? It's a very helpful tool and a great way to find calm and peace when you feel like so much is out of your control.

The following list of chakras and the accompanying issues is not at all comprehensive. If you're experiencing something that's not listed, first, I ask you to close your eyes and tap into your intuition. What is your inner voice telling you the issue might be linked to? Your body is very smart and will let you know what you need if you give it a chance to "talk."

You can also reach out to a respected healer...a shamanic practitioner, a reiki master, a Chinese herbalist, a nutritionist, a massage therapist, an acupuncturist, a yoga instructor, a qigong teacher, a midwife, your mother or grandmother, or a doctor. You can gain a lot of insight from seeking wisdom from many sources.

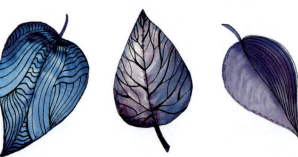

Table of Chakras
and Accompanying Issues

Root Chakra...Page 9: Training tip—love yourself.
Affects the immune system, enzyme activity, the fight or flight response, protein production, insecurity, depression, blood/bowel/bone disorders, anxiety, anorexia, obesity.

Sacral Chakra...Page 33: Training tip—connect with your inner child.
Affects the reproductive system, fat storage, water balance, genital/sexual/fertility issues and may cause joint problems, dehydration.

Solar Plexus Chakra...Page 61: Training tip—own your power.
Affects the digestive system, blood sugar balance, and can make you hypercritical, arrogant, or make it difficult to understand or control emotions.

Heart Chakra...Page 79: Training tip—have an attitude of gratitude.
Affects the lymphatic system, circulation, heart, lower lungs, and may cause you to dismiss unconditional love. It is bruised when you suffer heartbreak.

Throat Chakra...Page 105: Training tip—dream big.
Affects chewing, metabolism, hearing, sense of smell, speaking, thyroid gland, and may cause us to mask ourselves.

Third Eye Chakra...Page 123: Training tip—take action.
Affects mood balance, sleep, thought processing, brain activity, and pituitary gland.

Crown Chakra...Page 143: Training tip—open up to divine goodness.
Affects the nervous system, pineal gland, energy meridians, circadian rhythms, the body's ability to cleanse itself. May cause disorientation and limited conscious thinking.

"Let us run with endurance the race that is set before us."

— *Hebrews 12:1*

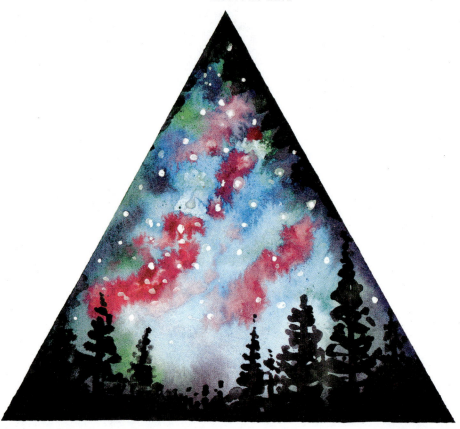

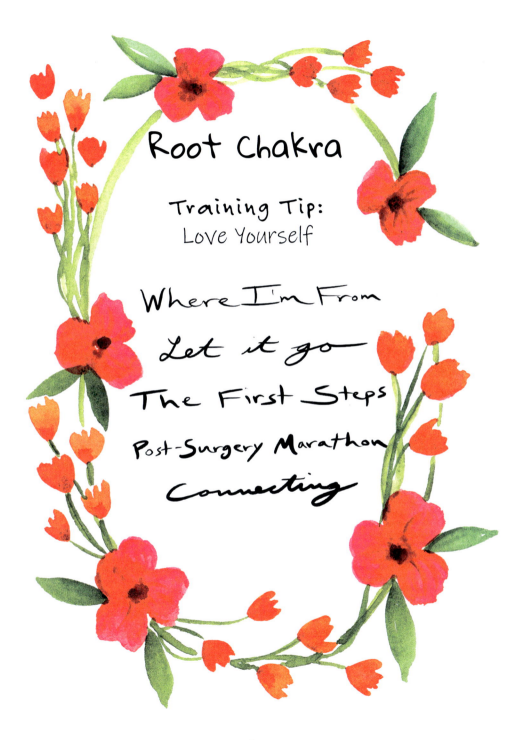

Root Chakra

Training Tip:
Love Yourself

Where I'm From

Let it go

The First Steps

Post-Surgery Marathon

Connecting

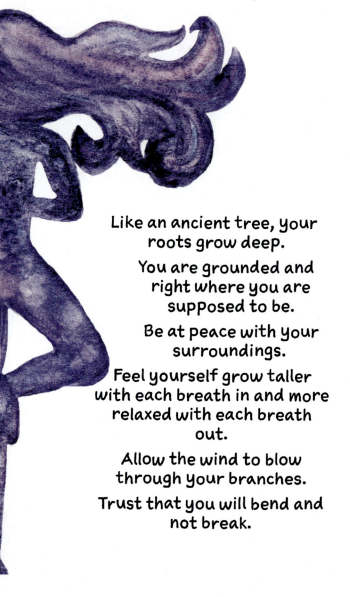

Like an ancient tree, your
roots grow deep.

You are grounded and
right where you are
supposed to be.

Be at peace with your
surroundings.

Feel yourself grow taller
with each breath in and more
relaxed with each breath
out.

Allow the wind to blow
through your branches.

Trust that you will bend and
not break.

Where I'm From

I was born in Morris, Minnesota, and moved to Zumbrota at six months old. I spent the first seven years of my highly imaginative life in Southern Minnesota.

Flickers of memory from that time include coloring all over the walls with permanent marker the day we moved out of a rental house, thinking I saved a baby bald eagle from the lawn mower in my front yard, playing Teenage Mutant Ninja Turtles with my three siblings (with my dad sometimes hopping in as Shredder), talking to the TMNT through manhole covers, truly believing I could fly like Tinkerbell—trying over and over again to jump off my bed and remain in the air—stealing gum from the grocery store—trying to hide the wrappers in the recycling bags—and having to return, apologize, and pay for the gum when my mom uncovered the situation (she's still a pretty good detective), playing hospital with my siblings and flying around the house with our little brother plastered with bandages and strapped to my dad's oil changing roller thing, covering my hand in glue, letting it dry, and peeling it off on the floor behind my dad's chair in the living room, learning how to ride my bike, losing our first family pet (our beloved black lab, Jamoch), bringing in our new yellow lab Bucky for show and tell, spraining my ankle on the teetertotter at school, hanging upside down on the monkey bars for the first time, having a teacher tell me he could connect my freckles like constellations and feeling completely embarrassed, thinking the Mayo Clinic was where they made mayonnaise, asking a lot of questions, sharing a room, riding the zip line my dad built (or maybe my brother did without him knowing) from the deck to the playhouse, watching my mom carefully pick tiny rocks out of my dad's torn-up, bloody legs and behind after a bad bike accident, and packing up our house and moving to Duluth the summer before third grade, where my parents still live and where I love to visit.

My imagination continued to serve me well when we moved. I continued to share a room. Now that I think of it, I've only *not* shared a room for two years out of my entire life. I think that in itself teaches you how to endure! I remember a lot of arguments. My sensitive soul hated all the yelling. Now, as an adult with a family of my own, I can only imagine the stress my parents were under. Moving to a bigger house in a bigger city, my dad starting a new job, four kids starting at new schools, trying to find their way, wanting to participate in many activities and sports that cost a lot of money, my mom starting to work full time as an art teacher, plus who knows what else. Anyway, I tried to block it out with my imagination...which I so often did with my best friend, Emily. We wrote plays, performed as talk show hosts, held fashion shows, played dress up with our younger brothers and her cat Freckles, tried to make coffee by crushing coffee beans and adding cold tap water, ate twenty-five-cent Little Debbie gas station snacks while watching *The Rosie O'Donnell Show*, created a secret fort in the woods between our houses, and enjoyed a pretty idyllic, easy-going childhood.

I'll never forget my third grade teacher, Mrs. Abraham. I loved her. We started every morning with the Pledge of Allegiance and singing "My Country, 'Tis of Thee" or "America the Beautiful" as she played the piano. I remember her smile, her joy, her warmth, her care for all of us. I remember sitting in a circle for class meetings where we discussed good news and problem solved. I remember writing almost every day in my blue spiral notebook (which I still have).

Looking back, my student teaching began in her classroom. Much of her persona and professionalism were deeply embedded in my psyche, and I now realize I carry on many of those same traditions. I wish I knew where she is today so I could thank her in person. If you're reading this, thank you, Mrs. Abraham. For everything. You are a hero of mine. During a big transition, you were such a guiding light.

My siblings and I started attending Minnesota Youth Ski League sessions at Snowflake Nordic Ski Center every Sunday. Because there were so many kids, we broke off into groups based on age. I didn't always love being out there, especially on the cold days. But we went regardless. I remember marking the kilometers we skied each week on a little chart so we could be proud of ourselves (and learn to compare ourselves to others, apparently).

I'll never forget the first race we did. Everyone else my age (or so it seemed) was skating, which is the faster of the two cross country techniques, resembling a more graceful hockey player. I was the sole classic skier, the traditional and much slower of the two techniques, where you glide in the tracks. I was frustrated when people kept zooming past me, so I hammered faster. Even though we all ended up with a ribbon, I know I earned it and it made all the fuss worthwhile. When I entered eighth grade, I began coaching the group and loved every second of it.

In Duluth, along the shores of Lake Superior and in the Boundary Waters, my wild heart began to take shape. Many of my most prominent childhood memories are from one camping trip or another, often in the great BWCAW, the Boundary Waters Canoe Area Wilderness, or simply Boundary Waters for short. It is a holy place in Northern Minnesota—a mecca of sorts for all outdoor enthusiasts. We took many trips there as a family. It was a place to escape reality. But what my parents taught us kids is that nature is our true, sacred, shared reality. I became best friends with the rocks, the water, the loons, the clouds, the infinite stars. My older sister, Rachel, and I used to make little villages out of rocks and sticks and play "house" until it was time to eat a freeze-dried meal of spaghetti that my mom had homemade and freeze-dried herself.

From fishing off of giant boulders, floating down rapids between lakes, paddling for hours, portaging while swatting away swarms of blood-sucking mosquitoes, playing cards in the tent to pass the time while a storm rolled through, and simply surviving the elements in thin ponchos during a cold and snowy October trip, I was made stronger, tougher, more resilient. Those family camping trips...full of bickering and solitude, frustration and awe...made me who I am today. It's where I learned the most important life lessons, such as being prepared, hard work, appreciating the little things, respecting the natural world, learning my place in the circle of life, the power of silence and breath, persistence, the sacredness of family and shared experiences, how to love myself, and how to endure.

I am from long starry nights
Sitting around the campfire
Where stories are told
And memories are made

I am from sparkling snow
Falling gently to the ground
Covering the land
In a blanket of diamonds

I am from sit-down family
dinners
As our days unfold over
Big, steamy bowls of chili

I am from endless portages
Lugging canoes and heavy
packs
Through mosquito country
In the Boundary Waters

I am from lakes as still as glass
And white-capped waves
That crash wildly onto shore

I am from northern lights
Dancing and twinkling
On a clear, crisp north-country
evening

I am from talk-shows
Fashion shows
Songs
Plays
And more
Created in the highly active
imaginations of best friends

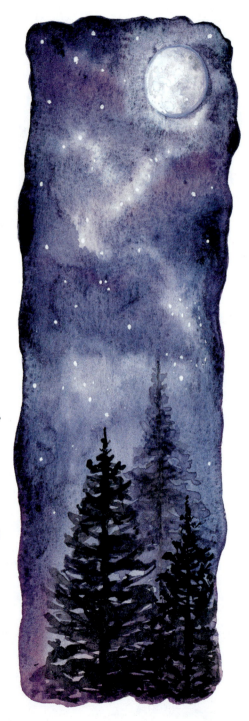

I am from Snowflake Nordic
Where the sun sets
Sending its rays of warmth and beauty
between birch trees and pines

I am from great-grandma's
Tupperware of sugar cookies
That are even sweeter
When made at the age of 102

I am from drying racks
Covered with socks, hats,
gloves
And other clothes smelling of
cold

I am from the crackling of
burning logs
In the woodstove
And the rustic smell it sends through the house

I am from the smile and endurance
of George Houland
The motivation of Dave Johnson
The heart of nature
And the endless love of all my
friends and family

Chandra Daw
October 27, 2003

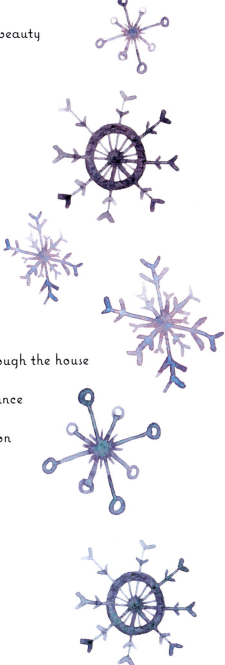

Let It Go

All right, since the training tip for this section is to love yourself, let's go there. One of the simplest things you can do to love yourself more is to let go of all that does not serve you. That's easier said than done a lot of the time, and what exactly does that even mean? For one, it means letting go of past baggage. As Elsa from *Frozen* sings, the past is behind us, we need to move on. Sorry, I can't help it. I'm a mom of three young girls.

I acknowledge that I had a pretty easy and privileged life growing up, but some memories I just don't need to remember—you know what I mean? It has taken time, but I've finally learned to forgive and move on. It's not like I forget. That's the hard part. Something will spark a memory or trigger me to react a certain way and I'll be like, "Well, shit, I thought I dealt with that." Healing the past truly is a lifelong process. Working through and letting go of truly traumatic experiences is a completely different story.

Let go of what others say or do that isn't for your greater good. Let go of gossip and comparison. Let go of anger, fear, bitterness, resentment, frustration, envy—all of that lower vibrational energy. It will take you nowhere. I take that back. It will take you somewhere. Down. It will take you down. You don't need that. You want to be lifted up. You need to surround yourself with people, experiences, work, music, and news that lifts you up. And most importantly...*you* need to lift yourself up with your thoughts and actions.

Self-care is such a buzzword these days in the workplace, in education, and on social media. You see it everywhere. And for good reason. I am privileged to live in a country and an era that encourages this practice equally for everyone. I am completely aware this encouragement is not true all over the world. It is a deep injustice. I wish that would change. It is one of my many dreams. However, I can only put my energy toward so many projects at one time. I'm choosing to focus on the here and now and, hopefully, bringing some positive change to you, dear reader...which will ripple out and affect countless lives.

What does self-care look like? It's simply loving yourself. Doing (healthy) things that make you happy, make you laugh, make you feel more relaxed and grounded, so you will be true to yourself, not take yourself so seriously, enjoy the little things, and have *fun*! This will look different for everyone. You need to find what works for you. You need to take care of you so you have enough energy to take care of others, to give to all the other areas of your life that need attending to, and maybe even to take on something new. You'll be happier and healthier when you do.

For me, one of the biggest self-care things I do is run. It's my natural high. I run at 5:00 a.m. I run when it's raining. I run with my kids. I run through the woods. I run when I'm happy, mad, sad, bloated, pregnant—anytime I can. I run in the best of times and worst of times. It's like a marriage. It's the solace I need in a busy world. It's where I ground myself with every *thump, thump, thump, thump, thump, thump.*

I'm not as consistent with running as my dear husband Erich. I swear he runs like a well-oiled grandfather clock (and he sleeps like one too). He runs (or skis) every day at 5:00 a.m. no matter what...no excuses. He keeps me going, that's for sure. When I don't run often enough, I get crabby with myself. Then I know it's time to kick it into gear again.

The First Steps

I like to say I began my journey as an endurance athlete and my "training" in my mother's womb. She won a ski race with me in her belly. I think that's a true story anyway. That's the fun thing about writing a memoir...a memoir is mostly memories...but with the freedom to take some literary license and add some flair when I feel the urge.

My parents skied with me and my three siblings in backpacks and pulks they handcrafted themselves long before the fancy Chariot, a multi-sport trailer and stroller, arrived on the scene. The contraption they created had long PVC-type tubes that attached to a plastic sled as well as a buckle that clipped around their waists. They would take turns pulling us kids, sometimes two at a time, so we wouldn't fall behind. It could not have been easy. But it was their desire and commitment to getting us outdoors and moving as a family that kept them going.

They had me on skis around the same time I started to walk. I have many memories of our times on the trail as a family—from the giant, hot pink fanny pack my mom wore that was stuffed with lemon drops, mints, and water to keep us all going to trying to keep up with my sister.

I continued my journey with endurance sports when I joined the middle school cross country running and ski teams. My older brother, Ben, and sister, Rachel, led the way. When I was in sixth grade, the ski coach, Dave Johnson, said, "I can't wait for you to be on the team!" That meant a *lot* to me as a tween trying to find myself. I loved every second of being a Duluth East Greyhound. The friends. The miles on the beautiful trails. The races. The spandex. All of it.

My little brother, Greg, did not follow the path we blazed. He went his own way. But he got back into endurance sports after high school. Once it's in your blood, you can't forget it. I remember doing our first race together, the first annual Duluth Duathlon at Lester Park. We ran three-ish miles on the trails, biked twenty-ish miles, and ran the same three-mile loop again to complete the course. I loved being able to compete with Greg. He went on to train for and complete many endurance events, including a full Ironman. He helped coach Northern Michigan University's women's track and field team for a few years and created the first collegiate mountain biking team in Minnesota at Lake Superior College in Duluth. I'm so proud of you, Greg. You've always been a trailblazer.

My high school running team won seven state championships. My sister was a part of the winning teams for several years (as was former Olympic runner, Kara [Wheeler]

Goucher). I had the honor of joining my sister and others as an alternate one year. I was also a part of the cross-country ski team. There were over 100 of us. On both teams there was a great mixture of athletes. Some trained hard with the hopes of making it to the state meet. Others were just out to have fun. All were accepted and part of the pack. I was a mix of both.

The Duluth East Greyhounds were a powerhouse for sure. We were also a pack. My teammates were my best friends. We trained together, ate lunch together, traveled together and went to prom together. I have so many memories from running the streets and trails of Duluth. To this day, when I go home to visit my parents and I'm driving around town, I can picture my teammates and me doing hill repeats up Glenwood Street or doing a ridiculously hard workout where we ran hard out Jean Duluth Road, sprinted up the never-ending hill of Pleasant View, and back to school.... Oh my sweet Jesus.... Or getting samples of ice cream at Baskin Robbins on Woodland Avenue before they closed, running, talking, and smiling with every step.

One memory that will be etched in my mind forever is from the winter of my eighth grade year. I'll never forget the team meeting we had in the basement of Snowflake Nordic Ski Center, where we practiced almost every day, year after year. I was one of the dozens of girls spread out around the dimly lit room anxiously waiting to hear what our coach had to say. Dave was letting us know who was going to be selected to compete at sections and state. There were a lot of really good skiers on our team, and as an eighth grader lacking self-confidence, I didn't count myself as one of them. In my heart, I knew I was. I worked hard, did all the workouts I was supposed to, and raced fast. But in my head, I had a laundry list of made-up reasons for why I wasn't worthy. Deep down, I had an ache to compete and prove myself. Turned out my coach could sense that desire. He picked me to join the ranks of the best skiers in the state over a senior. What? I was immediately flooded with a mix of emotions. *Oh, no, she's going to hate me. I don't deserve this. Why did he pick me? I can't believe he chose me. I did beat her in a lot of races. I*

feel so horrible about taking away her last chance to go to state.
OMG, I can't believe I'm going to state! I won't let you down.

That meeting was a huge milestone on my journey toward
believing in myself and owning my extraordinary endurance.
Dave saw something in me that I hadn't yet found. Perhaps
it was the sparkle in my eye or my game face at the start of
a race. He believed in me enough to give me a chance over
a girl who wouldn't get another. The gravity of the decision
weighed heavily on my heart, but truly made me feel weightless.
I emerged from that basement with a renewed vigor and
determination to step into my power, to test my limits, and to
tell *my* story through every stride.

The Minnesota State Championships were always held at
Giants Ridge in Biwabik. The memories I made there over the
years will stick with me forever—the piles of people huddling
together passing the time before their races, the matching team
spandex, the palpable nervous energy, the bunk beds, the pep
talks, Double Trouble and Triple Threat (aptly named sections
of the trail that were challenging to say the least), zooming
down the classic course after a monstrous effort in the first half,
the friendly rivalries between individuals and teams, the award
ceremonies.

My sister Rachel earned five individual state championship
titles in Nordic skiing and was selected to the Midwest Junior
Olympic ski team as well. She is amazing. As an athlete,
sometimes I felt like I was in her shadow. I sometimes felt I
could not fill her shoes when she left for college and I had two
years to live up to the legacy. But truthfully, I felt so lucky to
have her as my sister. She was my hero, and I loved her beyond
words. I still do. She went on to compete in both running and
skiing at Northern Michigan University, and made a name for
herself there as well. There isn't enough space here to write
about all her incredible accomplishments.

College Days

I graduated from high school in 2002, and went on to Gustavus Adolphus College (GAC) in Saint Peter, Minnesota, where I competed in cross country running and skiing. I was never as good as Rachel, but I tried my best, and it brought me joy (and a lot of pain—it's all a part of the process).

My Gustie teammates hold a very special place in my heart. There's something to be said about sharing a common pain. Many of us are still very close and get together at least once a year at the American Birkebeiner, or Birkie for short. The Birkie is the largest and oldest ski marathon in North America. The race itself travels 50-55 kilometers from Cable, Wisconsin to Hayward, Wisconsin. If the Boundary Waters is the mecca for outdoor enthusiasts, then the Birkie is the mecca for cross country skiers. Tens of thousands of skiers flock to the Hayward area every year to test their limits.

We love reuniting every year for the race. It's a goal that gets me out the door on frosty mornings. But for me, it's not about how well I do; it's about the electric energy I feel when surrounded by thousands of snazzy spandex-wearing skiers, the camaraderie, the stories, and the post-race celebration. We've been there for each other through so many of life's ups and downs— weddings, miscarriages, births, deaths, loss of jobs, new homes, promotions, and everything in between. The miles may separate us, but real friendships endure.

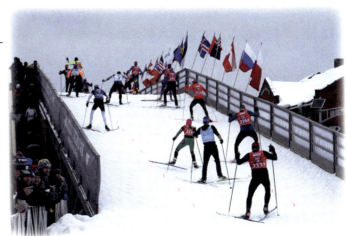

Me, in the green suit, skiing up the famous Birkie Bridge before racing to the finish line. February 2020.

On a recent run, I was reflecting on my days of pounding the trails in Southern Minnesota, not too far from where I first began walking. I thought about all the lessons I had learned on all the trails I had traveled. One of the greatest lessons came during a bounding workout my first year at GAC. If you don't know what bounding is, imagine a deer bounding over fence after fence after fence. Now imagine a person doing that with ski poles in their hands.

I had the longish van ride to Seven Mile Creek to let the butterflies get me all worked up and make me feel nauseous from thinking about the killer workout we were about to do. First year skiers only had to do five circuits (which was a super-hilly, horrible out and back trail). Everyone else had to do seven. I'm kind of guessing on the numbers—it may have been more. So, if you were too slow, you'd drop off the back of the pack and get to see your teammates essentially lap you! I was all sorts of nervous. I didn't know if I was up to the task.

We started with our warmup and all was well. We were talking, having a good time, and enjoying the view. It was indeed a beautiful trail. Then the bounding began. I tried my damnedest to keep up with the pack. It was hard as hell, and I wanted to throw up the whole time. Being the person I am, I told myself I was going to do seven circuits. "If they can, so can I!" But when I got done with the fifth, I hunched over my poles and told my coach, Scott Jerome, "I can't do any more.... I think I'm done." He could've said, "Great job, Chandra. You did great." Or "Really, Daw, that's all you've got?" Or "I know you can do more." But he didn't. He just stared at me, looking disappointed (maybe he wasn't, but in my freshman eyes, that's what I saw).

The truth is, he didn't have to say a word. I said it *all* to myself. *You suck. Why can't you just do two more? Maybe collegiate skiing isn't for you. You were never as good as your sister. Way to quit.*

I spat on the ground, dug my poles in hard, stared harder back at my coach, *I'm not a quitter; I have what it takes, just you watch*, and set off to complete two more loops.

It was miserably hard.

I probably cried, and I probably got a few blisters. But what I *know* I gained was deep satisfaction and much needed self-confidence. Maybe I could do this college skiing thing after all. Maybe I could achieve more than I could imagine. I pushed myself past my comfort zone, over the edge, deep into the pain cave, and I survived. I grew stronger. I set my goals higher. I trained my butt off for years.

I never grew to love bounding. What skier does? But I grew to respect the effort it took to achieve all I wanted to achieve. I grew and learned how to talk positively to myself. My coaches from high school on knew the exact time and place and words to use when they chose to speak. They knew when to stay quiet and let me figure things out for myself. They were the best coaches one could ever have.

I finally tapped into my strength and belief in myself and truly owned my power. As a senior, I qualified and competed in the Division I Nordic Skiing NCAA Championships in Steamboat Springs, Colorado—while in the throes of student teaching, no less. I didn't have time to fly out early to acclimate to the altitude. I didn't have a team with me or a wax crew of five coaches. But I did have my family. And my awesome coach, Jed Friedrich. And Scott Jerome, my coach for the first two years in college. Scott was extremely influential in my life. At Steamboat Springs, he put his hand on my shoulder and said, "I knew you'd make it!" I still have a letter he wrote to me folded up in an old jacket pocket, along with a letter to myself listing my big goals.

On the day of the race, I certainly wasn't the fastest. It was humbling to ski with the fastest college athletes in the country. Holy crap. I did my best and gave my all. I crossed the finish line and collapsed and was escorted to the local hospital with dehydration and exhaustion. They poked my lifeless arms, I swear twenty-five times, trying to find a vein. I watched my coach cry. I cried. I chugged down watered-down Gatorade. I was slightly embarrassed, but I bounced back from that ordeal and competed in the next event two days later. I don't give up easily. I may not be the first to the finish line, but I'm strong as fuck. I've always been a fighter, and I always finish what I start.

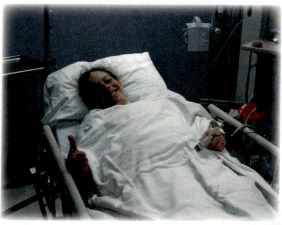

Giving my coach a thumbs up in a Steamboat Springs, Colorado hospital after the NCAA ten-kilometer classic race earlier that day. March 2006.

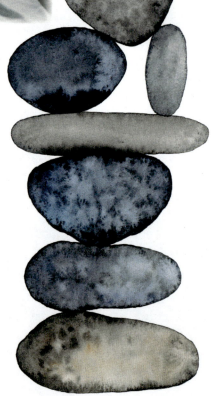

Connecting

Here are other ways I love myself, keep myself grounded, and connect with my root chakra:

- I go to yoga (well, I'm the teacher and kind of have to go…but I choose to teach, and I choose to show up). Even when the coronavirus took over the world and the center where I taught subsequently closed its doors, I still did yoga.

- I go to an energy class every week. Again, when we went into lockdown due to the virus, our conversations and meetings continued…albeit virtually, but they were still so very healing. The women in my energy circle are a big part of my tribe and rebirthed my passion for getting this book published. So, to them I say, "Thank you."

- I sit with a good book (or my journal or spirit cards) and a hot cup of coffee in the morning before anyone else wakes up.

- I drink a lot of water…most of the time. Other days, I drink way too much coffee and wine. It all balances out in the end.

- I let myself watch *This Is Us* and cry like a baby. (I know I'm not the only one.)

- I eat whole, natural, unprocessed, non-junkified food (90 percent of the time).

- I wake up and go to sleep with an attitude of gratitude and think positive thoughts.

- I forgive myself.

- I use Anchor essential oil and truly imagine that I am anchored to the Earth and present in each moment.

- I don't compare myself to other people or my family to other families. There's no point. We're all here to have our own experiences, learn our own lessons, and find out how awesome we truly are—just as God created us.

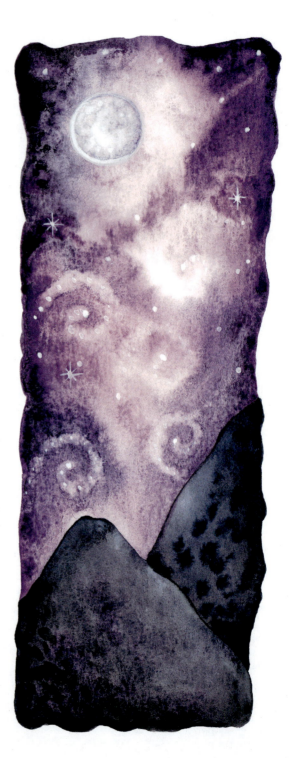

"The miracle isn't
that I finished.

The miracle is
that I had the
courage to
start."

— *John Bingham*

Chakra Guiding Questions

Root Chakra

Close your eyes, notice the sensation of your feet on the ground, and imagine roots from your feet growing deep into the earth. Check in with your root chakra. This is the energy center located at the base of your spine that connects to your sense of groundedness and survival instincts. When balanced, you feel stable, secure, full of health, energy, and vitality. How does it feel? Where do you think you are?

Do you love yourself enough?

_____

_____

_____

How can you love yourself more?

_____

_____

_____

Do you make time for yourself?

_____

_____

_____

How can you make the time?

_____

_____

_____

Where does your courage come from?

_____

_____

_____

If you don't have the courage or need a bit more, where can you get it?

_____

_____

_____

What would you like to start?

_____

_____

_____

What do you need to finish?

_____

_____

_____

NOTES:

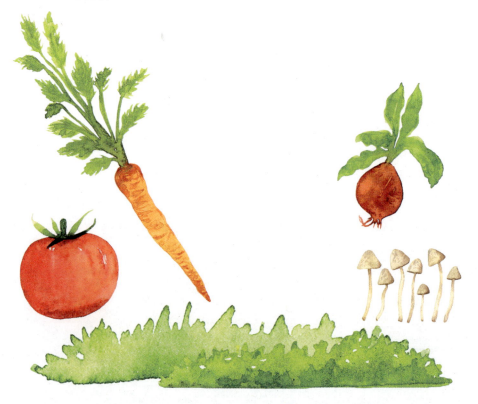

Chakra Training Tips

Root (Earth) Chakra

Visualization: As you inhale and exhale, picture a red lotus flower at the base of your spine, unfolding slowly. Breathe in and allow this warm energy to flow into your being. Breathe out and release your worries. Imagine the flower opening just a little more with each inhale and feel your body begin to be charged by a powerful source of energy.

Positive Affirmations: I am safe. I am secure. I am grounded. I am where I need to be. I am present and at peace.

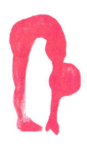

Crystal Therapy: Hematite, bloodstone, garnet, ruby carnelian, jasper, smoky quartz.

Wear as jewelry or just keep with you.

Nutrition: Dietary proteins, root vegetables, red foods.

Aromatherapy: Vetiver, Patchouli, Cedarwood. This chakra is connected to our sense of smell. Diffuse the oils, inhale directly from the bottle, or place a few drops on the bottoms of your feet.

Sound Therapy: Chant *lam* in the key of C or listen to thunder.

Yoga Poses: Mountain, Warrior One, Tree, Forward Fold.

Healing with Nature: Go for a walk outdoors and experience the sights, sounds, and smells. Sit on the grass under a tree and soak up the amazing earthly energy.

Remember, if you'd like more information about any of these healing modalities, you can check out the resources section at the back of the book. Namaste, friend.

Be Extraordinary

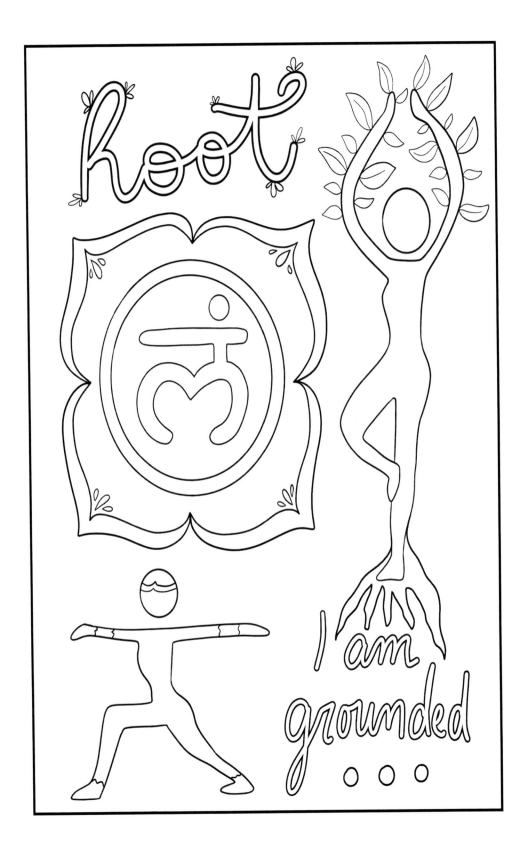

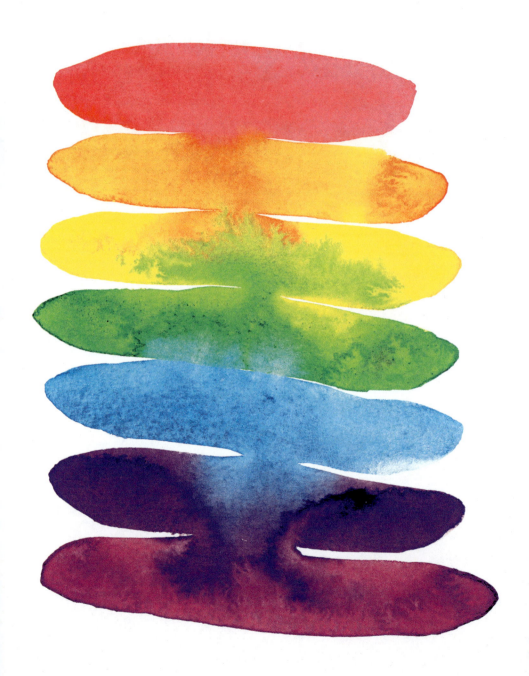

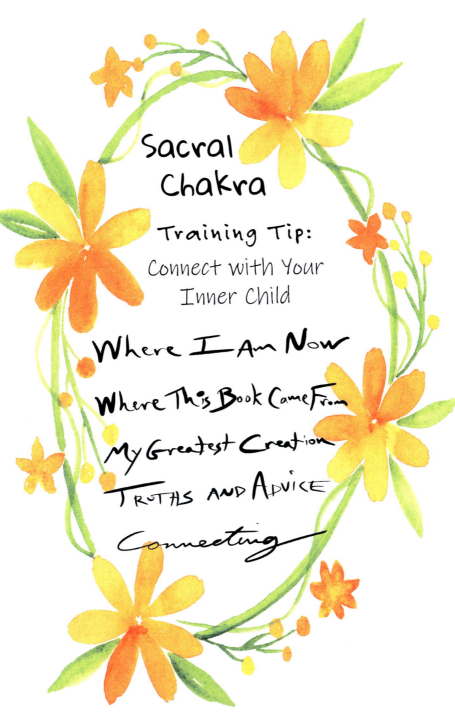

Sacral
Chakra

Training Tip:
Connect with Your
Inner Child

Where I Am Now

Where This Book Came From

My Greatest Creation

Truths and Advice

Connecting

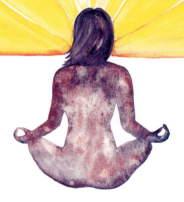

You are a unique and creative being.

You are connected to the source of divine creativity and radiate that bright light from within.

Where I Am Now

Right after graduating from Gustavus, I married my best friend, Erich. We've been married for almost fifteen years. We have three daughters: Emma is nine, Hali is six, and Kate is three; and two dogs: Keneu is thirteen and Fischer is six (also female). I pretty much married a saint. We live in a small town in the Upper Peninsula of Michigan. There's beauty to be found in every season. We get a *lot* of snow. We are cross country ski enthusiasts, and are blessed to have ski trails right outside our front door. We're pretty much in heaven during the long winter months.

Now is so momentary and seems to be ever-changing. As I'm writing this, I teach second grade and have been teaching for fifteen years (most of those years were spent teaching kindergarten). I coached cross country skiing at the collegiate level for one year. I've been coaching track and field for ten years, and it's a total joy to coach kids through a nonprofit I started called Iron Endurance. I have also started an orchard and community garden. I once started a short-lived Feed the Pigs initiative in our school cafeteria to eliminate food waste and help local farmers. I was so excited about it, and so were the kids. But I quickly discovered how hard change can be and how long systemic changes take to be fully implemented.

I'm a Little Free Library steward and have "planted" three little libraries around town. Little Free Library is the world's largest book-sharing movement. Its goal is to build community, inspire readers, and expand book access for all. Things I am equally passionate about. The community helped build, paint, and set up one of the outdoor book boxes at the Community Garden. Another is stationed at the ski hill in town. The third was also built and installed by

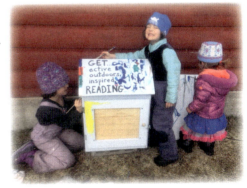

Emma, Hali, and Kate painting another Little Free Library. March 2020.

volunteers at a local park. Imagining all the books being read by people of all ages, especially kids, makes my heart smile.

I live in a four-bedroom, two-bathroom, unpretentious house that needs quite a bit of work on the exterior and interior. We've lived here for thirteen years, and there still isn't trim where there should be. But I really don't care. I have many passions that require my energy and focus. I do a lot of things for a lot of people and tend to take on too much at the same time. Sometimes, I feel very overwhelmed. But most of the time, I look around my busy, loud, messy, colorful life and feel totally at peace. These are the moments I dreamed about, prayed about, worked hard to achieve, and manifested. For example, I have a very distinct memory of me finishing up a run around Hartley Nature Center in Duluth and seeing two black labs, smiling and panting after a run with their owners, happily wagging their tails in the back of the car. I remember thinking to myself, *That's going to be me someday.* And here they are, happily dreaming away snuggled up together on one Duluth Pack dog bed (even though they have their own).

I get upset with myself for getting so frustrated about stupid things and having a short fuse. I feel annoyed when I can't even get two seconds to myself, and then I immediately feel guilty for feeling that way. (What the heck...do men feel this way, or just women?) I feel like something out there is calling me (like how Elsa feels in *Frozen 2*)!

Yeah, there's a lot going on in my brain at any given time. One of my energy friends once told me after smudging me with a bunch of sage, "Oh, honey, you're not grounded at all." And she laughed her Gina-esque laugh and added, "You're off in Chandra-land." No joke. In my head I was like, *Yeah, I know.... Wait, how does she know that?* Needless to say, I spend a lot of time on my root chakra.

Where This Book Came From

I'm a believer in stating your intentions and restating them until they're reverberating off every particle in the Universe. What you put out, you get back. Naturally, "write a book" was on the to-do list on my phone for years, but it's been in my heart for as long as I can remember.

I have dozens of journals, sketchbooks, scraps of paper, napkins, church bulletins, and pieces of a yoga mat (seriously) filled with ideas, feelings, poetry, stories, life moments, and randomness spilling off my shelves at home. But I didn't have a clue (or

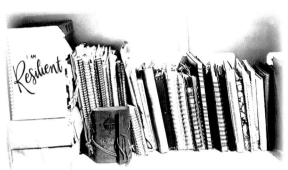

Just some of my journals.

maybe just didn't have the focus) to sit down and actually put all those ideas into any sort of order that would make sense to readers. Nor did I have a clue what the main idea should be. I think the major shift to making this book a reality started when I began paying attention to any sign from the Universe that was giving me direction and clarity for this book. Inspiration came in many forms: song lyrics, quotes, TED talks, children's books, shamanic journeys, spirit animals, and writing retreats.

The more I put the pieces together, the more I asked myself, *Why? Why do I feel so compelled to share? What lessons can I possibly give to the world?* I'm not an Olympic athlete or a famous person of any kind. I don't have any traumatic life-altering events I lived through. My custodian friends told me, "You're too young to write a memoir." Yes, I am still "young." But truly, age is just a number. I could be gone tomorrow and it wouldn't matter how old I was. And I'm pretty ordinary to tell you the truth. But what I've found in the telling of *my* truths is if you choose to give that little extra in life, you really are extraordinary.

With that feeling close to my heart and the knowledge that I could reach other ordinary people who were giving their own little extra, I wrote. If my daughters are the only people who read this, I'll be happy because I know they will use the message to continue to change the world for the better. But I'm a dreamer and a believer, so I *know* more people will pick this book up, read it, and be inspired.

I approached writing this book with unbridled energy and passion. It's for my girls, for all girls, for every single human who needs a boost of encouragement to live out their purpose and find the little extra they need. I hope my words reach deep into the crevasses of your heart and speak to the real you. Maybe the you whom nobody else knows. You know you. I know you. God knows you. You are enough. You are worthy of everything your heart desires. You are here for a reason. The world needs *you*!

Every single person has an incredible story to share. Mine is nothing special. I just listened to *my* heart, inner voice, higher self, the Universe, Mother Earth, God—it's all the same energy—and I knew I needed to share my stories, my truths with the rest of the world.

This book has many stories intertwined into one. Parenting, teaching, training, spirituality, and living my dreams, it's all me. I don't know how to untangle it. That's just who I am. Painting the masterpiece of my life one diaper change, one confident reader, one race, one prayer, and one story at a time, all takes extraordinary endurance.

At some point, you might ask yourself (as I did), "So, how the hell did you have time to write a book?" One answer is sacrifice. I sacrificed sleep. I woke up early before "the three littles" (our daughters) needed me. I stayed up late after the three littles went to bed. I sacrificed watching TV or checking social media or any other technological trap that's been created to distract us from doing what we were put on this Earth to do. I sacrificed exercise. I've been active my entire life, so sitting down to write was not always fun. While writing this book, I didn't work out as much as I was used to or would've liked to, and I felt guilty for wanting to write instead of exercise.

The other answer is I learned to connect with my inner child. When I was a kid, I wrote *all* the time, everywhere I went. It brought me so much joy! I wasn't doing it for anyone else. I did it for myself. I wrote to remember. I wrote when I wanted to connect with people. I wrote when I was sad and mad and glad and worried and confused and full of so many emotions I didn't know what to do so I'd just hold my journal and pen and cry onto the blank pages. The tear marks told their own stories.

I never lost my love for writing. It was always there, like an old friend. My journal was someone I could talk to about anything when I felt no one else could ever understand. As an adult, I returned more and more frequently with increased passion to my notebooks and my writing. I continued to be a mom, wife, teacher, coach, and everything else, but I started to put more and more energy into the written word. It brought me back to my childhood bedroom, my hideout in the backyard, my favorite tree in the Boundary Waters, and I felt at home. I felt alive. I *knew* this was what I had to give that little extra to.

Writing is a form of creating, full of raw, honest emotions that flow from the heart, through the pen (or keyboard), straight onto the paper. It is just one of the many ways to let yourself be creative and fire up your sacral chakra.

My Greatest Creation

The sacral chakra is connected not only to our creativity, but also to our sexuality and our reproductive organs. So, I'm going there next. You know what else I created that I'm most proud of? Okay, my husband Erich and I created them together…I couldn't have done it without him—love you, babe. We created our three beautiful children.

Being pregnant, having children, and being a parent is such a wild and exhilarating and rocky ride that requires such extraordinary endurance. I love my kids with every fiber of my being.

Kids, if you're reading this, I love you. When it comes down to it, that's all that matters. Love. Remember that as I go on a little trip down memory lane.

Our daughters are not babies anymore. But I discovered this journal entry from when Hali, our middle child, was an infant and felt compelled to share it in this space. My little angels came from a sacred space. And this was written, all of this book is written, from the energy deep in my sacral chakra. So here it goes.

Caution! If you are thinking of becoming pregnant or want to start a family, take this short quiz first. If you are already pregnant, take the quiz anyway to see what you're in for.

1. How many disposable diapers do you think you'll change in the first two months of your baby's life?

    a. 50

    b. 100

    c. 200

    d. None, I'm going to use cloth diapers

The right answer is E, none of the above.

Okay, that was a trick question. As I sit here in the dark at 5:15 a.m. writing this, with my nine-week-old swinging in the swing in the living room and my energetic three-year-old daughter sleeping in the twin bed that I just crawled out of in my infant's room and a cup of coffee to my left, I can honestly tell you I have changed well over 300, probably closer to 400 or more diapers. And that's trying to remember with my fuzzy, hormonal, post-baby brain.

Please, don't get all judgy on me or think, *Oh, how terrible of her,* because it's true. It's a simple fact, reader. Yeah, putting that number down in writing makes my incredibly eco-minded, carbon-footprint monitoring, nature-loving, environmentally-friendly conscience want to slap myself to Saturn and back, but there's just no getting around it.

To make yourself feel better about this fact, you can do what my husband and I did before our first child was born and plant dozens of trees to offset the hundreds of diapers going into a landfill. I know it's not much and we need to plant more, but at least it's something good to offset the bad. Or you could also use cloth diapers for as long as possible. We used them with our first child for over a year; then we had had it. Seriously, there is only so much poop cleaning two, let alone one, can handle.

2. How many times will you wake at night to feed your newborn?

   a. Two

   b. Three

   c. One

   d. None

The answer again is E, none of the above.

If you chose one of those, you're in la-la land and need to do a gut check. The truth is every child is different. That's what the parenting books will tell you. Well, we all know that, but what those books don't tell you is that it's completely possible to be up all night long.

Yes, you read that right, dear reader. Whether you are a woman who wants to get pregnant, a mom-to-be, a friend or family member looking to find a gift for a mom-to-be, or an incredibly supportive husband or partner, you (or they, depending on who's reading this) will have sleepless nights.

That's another fact. In the early, early days, you could be up every half hour and get maybe a total of an hour of sleep in between. If that math doesn't add up, I'm not going to apologize because a. I'm not a mathematician, b. I would still consider myself sleep-deprived, c. my brain is not fully functioning due to hormones and other factors, and d., simply put, I'm a mom of two.

The point is you will be up a lot. So try to get your mind wrapped around that. Or maybe it's better to stay in la-la land altogether. I'm not sure what the right answer is for you.

As a result of these sleepless nights, you may start to think you have a split personality. Just last night (I should really say morning) as I sat in the glider, baby in arms, staring into her beautiful wide eyes after nursing her, I was singing the song "Angels Among Us" in my head. I couldn't get over how beautiful and perfect she was with her adorable grin and baby noises.

Just a few weeks ago, this same scene played out quite differently. I sat in the glider, baby in my arms, staring into space after nursing her for the umpteenth time. I wasn't singing any sweet, angelic song. Instead, I was swearing under my breath, "Keep the fucking nukie in your mouth and go to bed!" and vowing that I was done having kids.

3. When your precious pumpkin grows into a toddler, your new favorite show will be?

a. The Voice, as it always has been.

b. Whatever show you like that's on at 8:00 p.m.

c. PBS (or some other kid-friendly network)

d. None. I don't watch TV

The answer is C.

If you said D, get over yourself and your altruistic ideals. I'm all for limiting TV and screen time in general. In fact, Erich and I were completely fine with the fact that we didn't have the capability when we bought our first house. It was my father-in-law who brought us into the twenty-first century so he could watch the news when he and my mother-in-law came over for dinner. I didn't even have my first cell phone until I was twenty-two. That's right, twenty-two. And even then, it was just a flip phone that had buttons with numbers on it so I could call people to talk to them. I now (at the age of thirty) have a smartphone. The point is, reader, that whatever your favorite show is, it will be no longer. Maybe it could be if you wanted to stay up late and watch it online or watch old episodes on the weekend, but you will soon come to realize those aren't great options for your health. You don't need me to tell you that you need sleep and you should spend your weekends doing things with your family that will create positive, lasting memories. Back to your favorite show—8:00 p.m. may be primetime in TV land, but it's bedtime (or dealing with post-bedtime drama) in toddler land. 'Nuff said. *Sesame Street* or any cartoon will become your saving grace when you're trying to do a million things. Trust me.

4. How long will a four-hour road trip take with a baby?

a. Four hours

b. Six or more hours

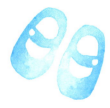

c. Five hours

d. Not gonna happen

The answer is B.

D could be an option if you want to remain a hermit until your baby grows up. You will have to make some adjustments and compromises, but if you'd like to maintain an active life and still visit loved ones, be prepared for things to take longer. When we took our first trip to visit my parents in Duluth with our first daughter, it took us at least six hours. It typically took four, but between stopping to nurse twice and bathroom breaks, it took much longer. When our second child came along, that same trip took even longer. Now, I not only had to nurse the baby; we also had to deal with a three-year-old whose bladder didn't work like clockwork and who had to go when we didn't have to go. And when you live in the UP (Michigan's Upper Peninsula), or any other part of the world where you are blessed with miles and miles and miles of trees and rivers and lakes, you and/or your toddler will end up peeing on the side of the road eventually. That's the tradeoff.

Truths

Here are some other truths of parenthood:

- Your child might clog the toilet with wipes, which might lead you to spend more than $5,000 dealing with septic issues.

- Your child might poop under the vanity in your room after an episode at the dinner table.

- You *will* rise at 5:00 a.m. to a fully energized two- or three-year-old who wants something to eat immediately.

- You will feel little fingers pulling at your eyelids and whispering a line from her favorite movie ("Do you want to build a snowman?") fully aware that it's still dark outside and probably not even 6:00 a.m. But according to her, it's *wake up time*!

- If you have more than one kid, you will have to explain to your toddler why your newborn is constantly at your breast.

- If you're a hunter, you will want to sleep for four hours straight in the deer blind rather than try to get a deer.

- You will listen to your toddler talk/sing/whine/cry for the entire four-hour road trip! Unless you choose not to go on any trips and live in a bubble. In that case, you will listen to your toddler talk/sing/whine/cry for four-hour stints at home. Either way, get ready for all that joy.

Advice

- Rise as early as necessary to do some quiet reading or writing because you know you'll have zero seconds to do so during the day.

- Resist the urge to hit snooze and rise up to get a workout in to a. train for a marathon, b. burn off the calories from all the Halloween candy you stole from your toddler's pumpkin because you know she won't really notice, and most importantly, c. stay sane and be a better mom/dad, spouse, and person as a whole.

- Be happy with where you are and your decisions. For example, going back to work after having a baby and pumping sucks...do it as long as you can and then stop when you can't take it any longer. If you can't or don't pump, good for you. Be your own cheerleader; no one is going to give you a high-five, or a gold star, or let you pick from a treasure chest when you finally get your little one to sleep through the night.

- Take time for yourself to do something you enjoy— whether that's doing yoga, meeting a friend for coffee, painting, or going out for a run.

- Take any help offered.

- Give a massage; get a massage.

- Play now, clean later; at times your house will look like a tornado has torn through it, but don't fret and don't sweat. You may want to clean and tidy up, and at times, that's okay. If you have a lot of patience, you can even use it as a way to teach your toddler about responsibility, etc., or you can turn it into a game (beat the timer). I admit, it is nice to look at a clean, organized living room. It is nice not to stumble over twenty-seven stuffed animals or stub your toe on a pile of books or step in spilt milk. Other times, cleaning seems futile. Why go through all that work and expend so much energy trying to cajole your toddler into cleaning when the house will look the same again tomorrow night? When I'm in that "why bother?" mode, I think, *Thank God I'm married to someone who likes to have a clean house. He'll help take care of that.* Love you, honey.

- Continue doing what you love with your children.

- Find out what your children love to do and do it with them.

- Take a painting class.

Giving advice is so easy, isn't it? Also, looking back and reading that journal entry in a normal state of mind makes me realize just how awful, sarcastic, and negative I could be and how important sleep is for our mental health. Oy.

Fast-forward to a more recent story and you'll see that I am still far from perfect. I often need to remind myself to connect to my inner child and imagine how she might feel before I act or react.

One night a few years ago, I took myself *way* too seriously and handed out one too many lectures. I let the two older kids watch *Sofia the First* a little longer than they should have, which led to them being tired and cranky, which led to them not being so kind to one another in the bathroom while getting ready for bed. Does this story sound familiar to anyone else? I could've walked away, or used a nice, calm tone of voice, or remembered to have a sense of humor or have some empathy…all those great parenting and teaching tricks that I know work and I've used before a thousand times. Instead, my short fuse blew up, and I got irrationally upset. I'm an emotional one for sure. I wonder where the girls get all their drama from?

Anyway, once we all settled down and I got them to bed, I heard yelling and arguing, so I went *back* into their bedroom. They sleep together on the bottom bunk, which is a futon, and they were fighting about stealing covers or something of the sort. I looked at Emma, the oldest, who had a thousand things around her and said, "Emma, look around you! I just don't understand. Why do you need all this stuff?" And as I watched the tears well up in her eyes as she proclaimed, "It's just that I love you so much that I have to build up all this stuff around me to try to replace you and help me calm down!" I seriously melted. I embraced her and said how much I loved her and how happy I was that she still loved me even when I yell at her. We were able to rewind the not-so-good bedtime and end on a super lovey-dovey, peaceful, and calm note.

I don't like to complain. I like to focus on the positive. But I also just want to be real. Parenting is hard. We're all doing the best we can. Whether you're a parent of little kids, big kids, furry kids, or no kids, I know you can relate. You were once a kid yourself. Maybe this chapter will allow you to forgive your own parents or forgive yourself. Or thank them! We're all human. We make mistakes. Maybe it will provide you with a little peace of mind that you're doing okay. Maybe it will encourage you to stay grounded and live in the present moment. I hope it will help you endure whatever season you are in.

One of my favorite parts of being a parent (and I'm sure I speak for Erich too) is sharing our love for the outdoors and silent sports with our children. It's been such a blast watching them take to it and begin their own journeys. I'm not sure what the future holds for them, and I truly just want them to be happy. Whether they stick with endurance sports will be up to them, but for now, it sure has brought many wonderful memories and has helped lay a strong foundation for a healthy future.

While there can be many rip-your-hair-out moments as a parent, there are far more joyous moments and reasons to celebrate. Life in the present is such a tremendous gift. In fact, it is all we have. Children are kind, intelligent, incredibly sweet, far more enlightened than we give them credit for, and simply hilarious.

And because I always like to look for the pearl, I would like to end this chapter with a letter I wrote to Emma and then just a few of the wise and wonderfully uplifting words from our children. I hope they fill you with joy.

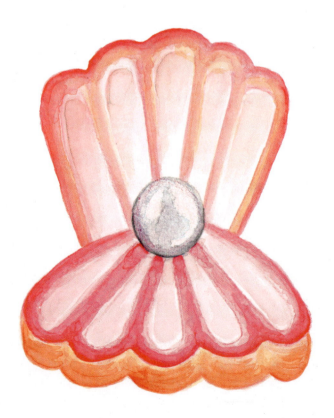

Dear Emma,

Watching you out the window today, I cried. I saw you. The most perfect you in all your creative beauty and artistic glory...paint, glitter, snow, mix, mix, mix, shake, spread.... "It looks like the universe!" you said. I saw you. The most helpful you carrying your baby sister, helping her with her rain boots that kept falling off. Then later, you quietly came into Kate's room as I was putting her to bed. You kissed her. Squeezed her tight and said, "You are so beautiful and kind! You will change the world. I just love you so much. You will make the world a better place because you're so kind."

The tears once again rolled down my cheeks. You noticed. "Why are you crying?" All I could squeak out was, "I just love you so much." But in my heart, I thought, Maybe I'm doing okay as a mom. Maybe the messages and lessons I'm trying to impart to my children are really sinking in. Because you know what, sometimes it's hard to tell if you hear what I'm saying. Like, how many times have I said, "Put your pajamas on, brush your teeth, that's enough chips, hands are for helping, stop hitting your sister...for God's sake!"?

There have been times as your mom that I thought I should've invented a remote with the same repeated phrases to save my mental health and voice. But tonight, while rocking Kate before bed and hearing you whisper such tender words, I can pause and thank God that the things I'm saying and how I'm living are having a positive influence. God bless your beautiful soul, Emma. I love you so much.

Love, Mom

Children's wise and wonderful words

"It doesn't matter what color you are. The most special thing is that you have someone who loves you."

"What matters the most is family, the world, and life."

"I am so thankful for me, you, and life, Mother Nature, my sisters, my family and friends, and my home."

"Your imagination will follow you wherever you go."

"I love you more than you know."

"You make my heart shine!"

"I know this is going to be scary, but I can handle it."

"I can do this. I just have to be brave."

"I will pray for you."

"My favorite part of life is to see you."

"I want to be just like you."

"I just want to snuggle."

"You're my best friend."

"I miss you all day long."

"I love you so much because your spirit is so beautiful."

"Do you have a voice? What do you want to talk to me about?"

"I will help you heal."

"Can you come sing me a sweet song? I can't fall asleep."

"Dream away."

"Go to sleep, go to sleep; you are my best friend; close your eyes; don't wake up, go to sleep; you are so precious to me."

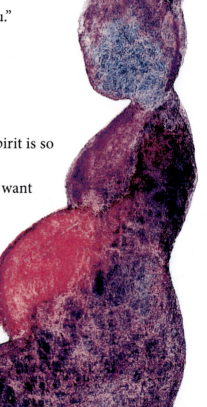

Post-Surgery Marathon

You could probably guess by now how I stay sane while juggling all my dreams and extra commitments, being a good wife, a mother of three girls, and a full-time teacher… running. I could add other things to the list for sure…skiing, biking, fresh air in general, writing, yoga, talking it out, my crockpot, wine. It all helps. But running keeps my body fit, my mind fresh, and my spirit flying free. I remained dedicated to running and skiing throughout pregnancy and motherhood for my sanity. I listened to my body and slowed down as needed. There were days I waddled more than anything, but I still moved. Remaining still would often leave me feeling stuck in any negative mood or moment. To carry on my mama's legacy, I'm proud to say I completed three ski races while pregnant.

I've toed too many start lines to count, but dear reader, I want you to know that it was not easy to get to this particular start line that I'm going to share with you. Six weeks prior, I was dry heaving into a garbage can in a hospital. I couldn't dress myself, do my own hair, or pick up my baby. I was in a lot of pain, feeling totally frustrated and out of control. I was a mess. The silver lining was that it could've been worse. That's always the truth. Having had the carpet swept from under my feet after training diligently for the Marquette Marathon with hopes of qualifying for the Boston Marathon, I had to make peace with the fact that I would not be able to move the way I envisioned myself moving or not be able to do it at all.

While I was hooked up to different machines wearing nothing but an airy hospital gown, feeling at my absolute worst, Erich whispered, "It's still a ways away…it's still possible…don't count yourself out." My husband knew what was going through my mind. I smiled (because that's what I do), but I thought, *He must be crazy.* Did he see me? Did he honestly believe I could come back from this and do a *marathon*? He did believe in me. Always has. Always will. He bought me a brand-new pair of running shoes to prove it.

Well, I did it.

I toed the line. I had no idea what those 26.2 miles were going to bring, but I was ready to pick up the pieces and go for it…. Because I was no longer broken (technically, I was still healing, but the doctor gave me the okay). Because we're made to test our limits. Because life is too short. Because I paid to do it and didn't want to waste the money. Because I have to finish what I start even if it ends differently than what I imagine.

Connecting

Other ways I connect to my inner child, source of creativity, and sacral chakra:

- Rocking in happy baby pose. It feels so damn good.

- Having faith like a child. I believe in all God's goodness and everything spirit-related with every fiber of my being.

- I love being creative…painting, drawing, writing poetry, getting crafty with my kids. I feel a deep sense of peace and connection to the infinite power of the universe when I do so.

- I connect through the eyes of my own children. Boy, it's like looking in a mirror sometimes. It's also like looking at the face of God.

- Tickle fights, airplane rides, underdogs, spontaneous dance parties, playing dress up, running barefoot through the grass, playing in our fairy garden, finger painting, laughing until I cry, and reading well over a thousand children's books a year.

- I'm an elementary teacher, so basically, I connect with my inner child every day. 😎

What a blessing it is to experience life through the eyes of a child yet have the wisdom to be able to guide them on their journey.

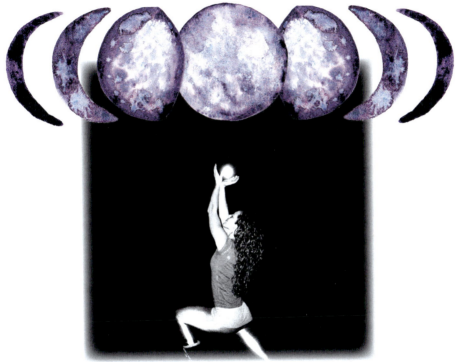

*Embracing the supermoon. Soaking in the
power. Feeling my creative spirit pulsing
through my veins. Ready to endure like a
warrior.*

"Yesterday is gone.
Tomorrow has not yet come.
We have only today.
Let us begin."

— *Mother Teresa*

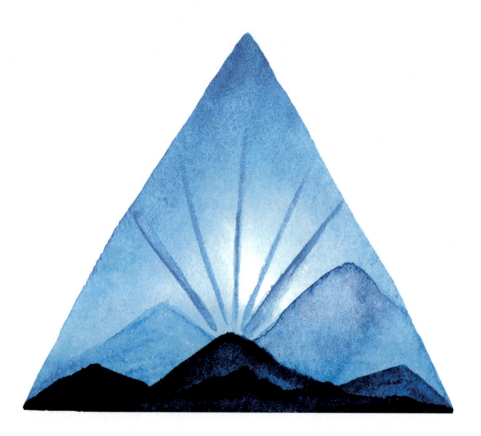

Chakra Guiding Questions

Sacral Chakra

Close your eyes and tune into the area of your body about two inches below your belly button. Check in with this sacred area, your sacral chakra. This is the energy center located in the reproductive area of your body that connects to your feelings, emotions, sexuality, and creativity. When balanced, you feel grace, flexibility, depth of feeling, sexual fulfillment, and creativity. How does it feel? Where are you?

Do you connect with your inner child?

_____

_____

_____

How can you connect more?

_____

_____

_____

What have you already "created" that you're damn proud of?

_____

_____

_____

What else do you want to create?

_____

_____

_____

What "yesterdays" do you need to let go of? Write them down on a separate sheet of paper; then light them on fire. Let that shit go!

_____

_____

_____

What "tomorrows" are you worried about? Write those down too and burn them.

_____

_____

_____

How will you live in the present today?

_____

_____

_____

NOTES:

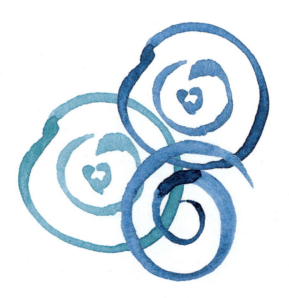

Chakra Training Tips

Sacral (Water) Chakra

Visualization: As you inhale and exhale, picture the orange of a risen sun just below your belly button reaching outward. Breathe in and stir the color counterclockwise. Breathe out and visualize the orange turning into a cone. Imagine bright energy flowing back through the cone with each inhale. Feel the flow of creative ideas and be filled with joy.

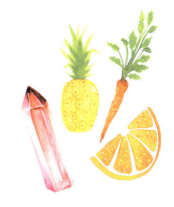

Positive Affirmations: I am a unique, sensual, and creative being. I attract whole and nurturing relationships. I am alive and connected. I feel radiant and beautiful. I embrace life with passion and joy. I will use my gifts to make the world a better place.

Crystal Therapy: Red and brown aventurine, red garnet, red jasper, carnelian.

Nutrition: Water, tropical foods, orange foods, fish.

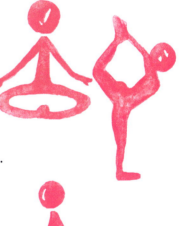

Aromatherapy: Jasmine, bergamot, clary sage.

This chakra is connected to the element of water. Use these essential oils in a bath or body scrub or place a drop on your temples.

Sound Therapy: Chant "*vam*" in the key of D; listen to the ocean or rainfall.

Yoga Poses: Dancer, triangle, cobra, butterfly.

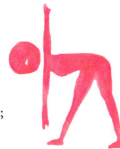

Healing with Nature: Spend time by or in the water; drink more water.

Be Extraordinary

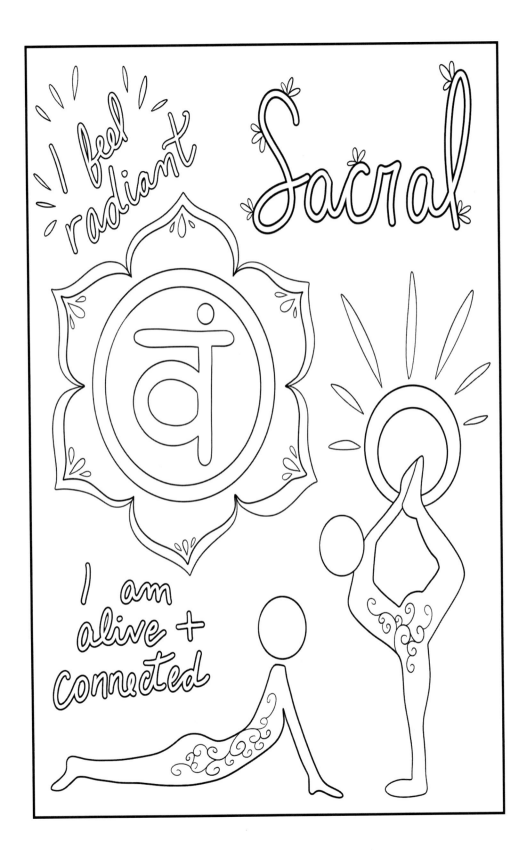

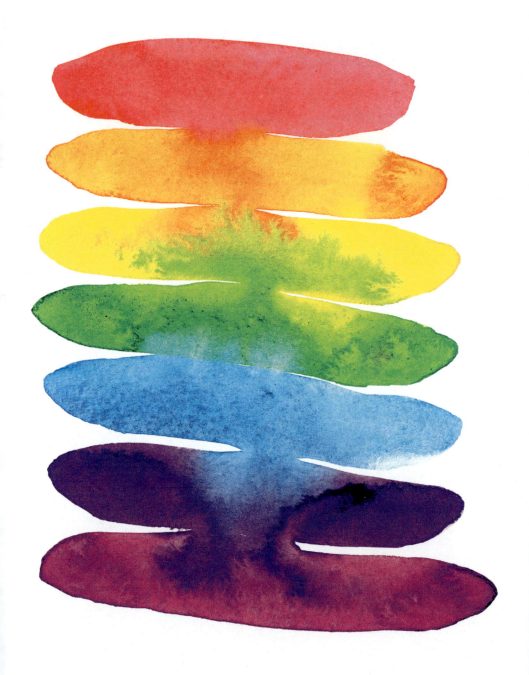

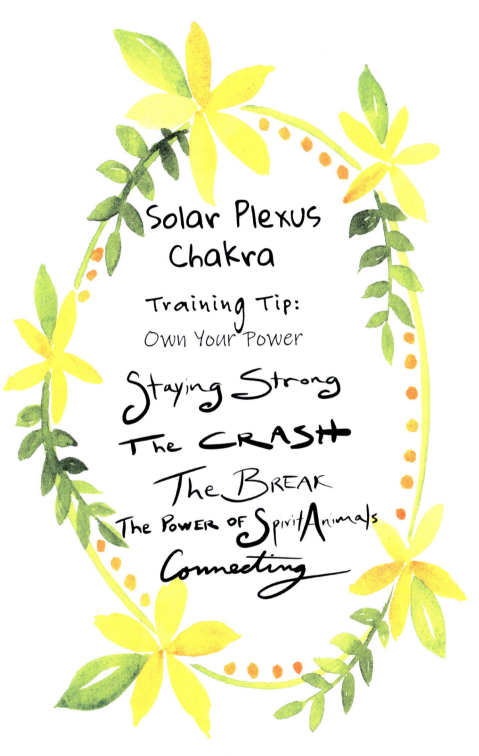

Solar Plexus Chakra

Training Tip:
Own Your Power

Staying Strong

The CRASH

The Break

The Power of Spirit Animals

Connecting

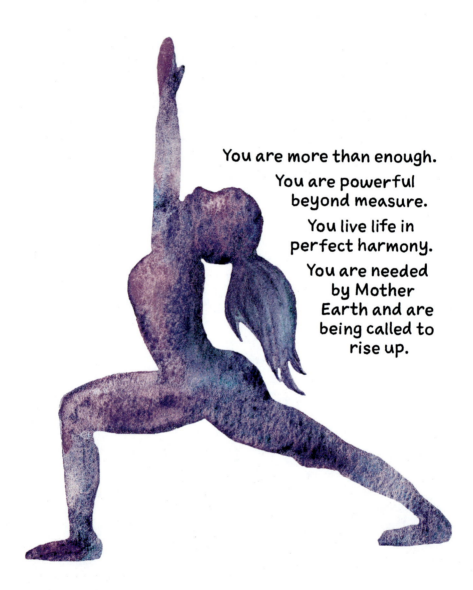

You are more than enough.

You are powerful beyond measure.

You live life in perfect harmony.

You are needed by Mother Earth and are being called to rise up.

Staying Strong

Running and skiing have brought me to places I wouldn't have otherwise gone. They have taught me lessons I wouldn't have otherwise learned. They have brought me lifelong friends and my wonderful husband Erich. Most importantly, being out on a trail has taught me how to endure pretty much anything life throws my way.

Running and skiing can transform lives. If you feel like giving either or both a try, I promise you won't be let down. I believe they will do just the opposite. They will lift you up! Just begin. Wherever you're at is okay. Keep putting one foot in front of the other. Run when you don't want to, and pretty soon, you won't want to live without it.

I realize how incredibly privileged I am to be moving at all. I am privileged to be *able-bodied*. I am privileged to have the ability to move my own two feet. I am privileged to go out for a run without fear of being questioned by police or enduring hateful racist speech. I am privileged to be able to afford the proper gear to enjoy endurance sports. I am privileged to be able to go out for a run and breathe in fresh air. I think about these things every time I lace up my shoes. I want to be as inclusive and welcoming as possible. I understand that many people have had to endure a *lot* more than me. There's a good chance *you* have endured a lot more than me. To you I say, "I love and bless you. You are a tremendous blessing. You are my hero. Keep enduring, dreaming, and finding ways to stretch boundaries—and stay strong."

If you are blessed with more, I hope you can find ways to give to others. Listen to your gut. What are you fired up about? What do you want to give a little extra to? Nonprofits abound that would love your help. May I offer my biased opinion? Public schools and children are always in need (and very appreciative) of donations. Perhaps you could donate nice running shoes. Or maybe you don't have a lot of extra cash but you're skilled in one area or another. Reach out to your local school and offer your time as a volunteer. Most teachers would be more than happy to have someone else come in and teach for an hour. And kids are always excited about something "different." All right, I'm getting a bit off topic. Time to focus.

I continue to be active because it's in my DNA. I don't know how to live without endurance sports. It gives me confidence and is a depression squasher. I've never been depressed, but I do get testy, moody, irritable, down on myself, and/or just plain down in the dumps when I don't exercise regularly. Staying active allows me to stay fired up about all my dreams and ambitions, which, in turn, gives my heart more energy to give to others. All the chakras are connected. When one is off balance, it affects others.

I once told Erich I was going to take a year off from training for marathons so I could focus on my writing. I even turned to prayer as well as my *pendulum* (which is connected to higher consciousness and my spirit guides) for a push in the right direction. At first, the advice I got from my Higher Power was, *You'll have a book published within a year if you just concentrate and put forth a more concerted effort.*

Okay, fine. So, I started writing more and working out less. I told myself I could make it happen. But then I felt the fire fizzling out. The internal flame that keeps everything else burning was fading. Not only was I not working out as much, but I wasn't writing as much either.

The truth is I didn't have enough energy, enough drive. I needed to exercise to feel energized. I needed to feed the flame. Honestly, I felt like I needed to take another go at qualifying for the Boston Marathon. It may sound completely ridiculous and totally crazy, but doing all that hard training gives me more energy, makes me more joyful, and more often than not, provides inspiration for my writing.

I know research out there attests to the cognitive and mood-enhancing effects of running and other cardio training. I truly crave the *flow state* during a run or a ski where everything else gets tuned out...even myself. I've had out-of-body experiences while on long runs, where I sense my true self, my spirit-self, looking down on my physical-self from above. I love feeling that complete disconnect from all the distractions of modern life and all the chatter in my brain. It is the feeling of being light and free and connecting with the earth under my feet and the air supporting my lungs. In that state comes enlightenment, self-realization, the ability to tune into other realities, and complete clarity.

But guess what? A few weeks after deciding I wanted to train for another marathon, I realized I needed to be home instead. If you can't follow that back and forth, it's okay. Erich has a hard time with it too. I don't know what it was. It's not like I heard God's voice saying, *"You must stay home with your family,"* or got struck by lightning, or had a vivid dream with a path laid out for me. No, it was simply that there were many "what ifs" and "who knows?" about the future. I decided I needed to conserve my energy and be an anchor for my family. And then do you know what happened?

The coronavirus.

Bam!

All of a sudden, Erich and I found ourselves at home with our three daughters beginning on March 14, 2020, and continuing for the remainder of the school year! As I sit here in the early morning at my grandpa's old desk, writing with a crazy rain/thunderstorm swirling around outside, the decision to reopen schools is also up in the air. *Now* I see why I needed to conserve my energy. Being a parent and a teacher (and a good spouse on top of that) 24/7 while socially isolated without a break from one another takes more endurance than anything I've ever experienced.

In hindsight, I can say that my clairvoyance was on point. I knew something big was coming. I knew I needed to stay strong in a different way. I was going to have to endure much. I found balance with running and being a mom. I lived in the present more than ever before. I was grateful for the opportunity to strip away the trappings of the world and just be. God forced us to find new ways of being and helped us endure. That is a different book altogether.

The Crash

A year before the pandemic, I was training for the Marquette Marathon to build myself up to try qualifying for the Boston Marathon. I was right on schedule—then I decided it would be fun to hit some mountain bike trails with a friend. I should've listened to that faint little whisper that said, *This is not a good idea.*

The single track was amazing. I was cautious, of course, but let myself soak in the magic of the flow. After almost two hours of riding, my friend said, "What do you feel like doing? There's one more trail we could try. It's up to you." I was tired and getting hungry. I should've said no, but in my head, I thought, *I'm probably never going to come back here again. I might as well do it now.* "Let's do it!" I said.

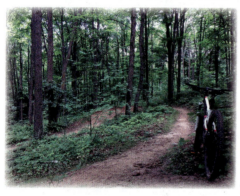

It was such a fun, fast trail, and all was well until I followed my friend over a little berm.

I hesitated.

Big mistake.

I barreled over the front of my bike and put my hands out to catch my fall. Another big mistake. I knew instantly that I had broken my collarbone. I sat there in a ball, helplessly trying to hold my shoulder up, getting eaten alive by mosquitoes because I wasn't even able to swat them away. And then I had the nerve to reach up and touch my collarbone.

Fuck!

I don't think I even cried. I was probably in shock. My friend came back, and thankfully, someone was doing maintenance on the trails—in the middle of nowhere Wisconsin—who drove the four-wheeler/golf cart/work machine to where I was to bring me back to the parking lot. That bumpy ride back was the worst. My friend then drove me about two hours to the hospital.

Erich met me at the hospital in Iron Mountain, Michigan. As we walked through the emergency room doors, I caught my reflection. *Wow, Chandra. Way to go.* I sat down in a waiting room chair, and guess what? I waited some more. During all the waiting, I let myself get really negative. I blamed myself. I said some really mean things. All internal, of course. I stewed and stewed. It was not pretty. *What the actual hell! Why did you decide to go biking? You did this to yourself. You did all that hard training for nothing. Why do you have to be so dumb? How much is this going to cost? You're so selfish. Way to ruin your chances of running Boston. Now you'll have to wait another who knows how many years.* And on and on. What was going on in my head matched exactly what I looked like on the outside—ripped up Lycra bike shorts, dried, crusty blood trickling down my leg, muddy, bloody face, smashed-up lip.

Then I had to endure the emergency department doctor who, after asking an ungodly number of questions and somehow discovering I don't eat dairy, told me maybe I should drink more milk. As if *that* was the reason I broke my collarbone. What the hell? In the end, I learned that I broke my clavicle in four places. Then, after a week of extreme pain and more waiting, I had surgery to put in a plate and seven screws.

The Break

I've certainly had my challenges through the decades—none insurmountable or extraordinary, but challenges nonetheless. We all have challenges. It's a part of learning and growing. However, I had never broken a bone before. And before the accident, I had never been without my silent sports for more than a few days, let alone twenty-five. That kind of sounds ridiculous and trivial, and I don't mean to sound like a whiner, but breaking my collarbone sucked. I've never sat in as much stillness as I did in the month following my crash. I could not even envision myself enduring so much stillness simply to let myself heal. It was not in my plan, dammit! It was eye-opening and liberating and momentarily blissful, but also incredibly frustrating, and at times, simply unbearable. Running (skiing, biking) is more than just exercise to me. It's my friend, my therapy, my motivation, my meditation, my prayer.

Yes, I made myself sit still and heal. I listened to the doctors (and others as well). I'm not that stubborn. I appreciated all the love and strength from everyone's positive thoughts and prayers, cards, visits, and meals. They truly helped. I also rallied vast energy and healing from various spiritual paths and alternative medicines...*everything* helps! I iced. I napped. I prayed. I meditated. I read. I walked a little. I snuggled. I laughed. I sat with my Tibetan prayer flags and let my shit go with the wind. I did a little yoga. I went on a shamanic journey calling on the strength and guidance of spirit animals. I ate healthy. I took my vitamins. I used oils. I drank plenty of water. I journaled.

Then finally, one morning, I woke up and said to myself. "I can't take it anymore! I need to go for a run." I felt like I could crawl out of my skin. I needed to go. So I did three slow, steady, sweaty miles. It was heaven. I was back in my element, listening to my heart without judgment. I got out of my own way. The spiral of dark, counterproductive thoughts drifted away with the clouds. I intentionally took back my power and regained my strength one step at a time.

The Power of Spirit Animals

On my slow trod down the road, I noticed several animals who seemed to be speaking to me. Having been enlightened to the power and timing of spirit animals and the messages they hold, I did not take these sightings for granted. Of course, I went back to my newfound "beastie" of a book, *A-Z Guide to the Illuminating Wisdom of Spirit Animals* by Sarah Bamford Seidelmann, and read about the animals. The story of how I came to own this book is a miracle in itself. And the book has been a huge help on my journey of healing and living my best life.

I was in Duluth visiting family. My brother Greg and I went for a sixteen-mile run on the Superior Hiking Trail. (Yes, it was as beastly as it sounds but also tons of fun.) Our amazing mom drove way out of town to pick us up with a cooler full of drinks and snacks, so we didn't have to do an out and back. She's the best. Later that day, I met up with some of my closest friends, my sisters, Megan, Mary, Cory, and Anne at the Amity Coffee Shop. There was a pile of books in the back next to some comfy chairs. I checked them out as I waited for my drink. I picked up Seidelmann's book and immediately knew I had to have it. As I hugged it against my chest, I looked up and read a sign on the wall, "*Feel free to take a book if it speaks to you.*" You couldn't wipe the smile off my face. As it turns out, that sixteen-mile run with my brother would be my last long run for quite some time. The serendipitous timing of the book finding me was not a coincidence. That was purely divine intervention.

On my first run post-surgery, I saw one loon calling in flight right above our house, five deer, two foxes, and a turkey feather!

Seidelmann says, "Loon has a fierce spirit of dedication to help you work through any challenges you face." Yes, I do. I am fierce when I need to be, so look out, world! I couldn't sit still any longer. I would not let a broken collarbone stop me. I would reclaim my power and rededicate myself to my training and all my passions.

Where I live, it's not uncommon to see many deer while out running. They're all over the place. However, on this particular afternoon, they seemed to be sending me a message. Deer appear to remind us that "Hurdles can now be cleared." Yes, they can. Yes, I can! Thank you, deer. Thank you, Sarah Seidelmann.

Seidelmann, also a shamanic healer, says, "Fox trots mindfully into your life and invites you to consider a more powerful alternative: just trusting your own instincts and acting on them." Without hesitation, I acted on my instincts to go for a run. They were animalistic in nature. Fox let me know how spot on I was with my need to get my ass moving.

According to Seidelmann, my soul sister-friend whom I will meet someday, "Turkey reminds us to breathe…it is a privilege to be alive to roll in the dust and to soak in the sun. Turkey does not waste time worrying about the past or fretting about possible outcomes." Yes, yes, yes! One-hundred percent. Turkey carries ancestral wisdom and reminds me that "dancing in your own eccentric style comes naturally." Amen, turkey friend! And thanks again, Sarah. Your book is such a treasure and helpful guide.

It's not like I thought I'd be back on track to qualify for Boston after this run. I wasn't even sure I'd be able to toe the line at the Marquette Marathon. But then again, I told myself, "Never say never." I was happy just to be running again (even though it was only one day).

Life can throw you curveballs, and having something to fall back on can give you incredible strength. That strength and motivation are critical to healing and allowing you to follow your passions, wherever they take you (in glorious pursuit or simply to stay sane). My something is running. After this run, I was happy to say my silence from silent sports was over—still no longer. Thank God!

Connecting

Here are other ways I own my power and connect to my solar plexus chakra:

- I am comfortable with myself, and although I classify myself as a major introvert (I am a true cancer, moon child), I am comfortable with others. This means what others do and say does not bother me in the least. This took time to hone, let me tell you. I used to take things way too personally. Now I'm like, *Hmm, that's nice,* or *Hmm, oh, well,* or *Hmm, you're acting like a complete jackass, but that's your karma, not mine.*

- I do enough core strength work to keep the area of my solar plexus chakra strong, fired up, hot, and ready for action. I say enough because I used to be crazy about it. Now, I might drink a little too much wine and might not do enough ab work to compensate for that. But now I'm like, *Hmm, oh, well. I feel strong enough.* When I get super fired up about training for another marathon, I'll probably get a little more serious.

- I know what I'm in control of and what I have no control over. I don't waste energy on the latter. Thus, I remain power*ful* rather than power*less*. And please let me clarify…I don't mean power as in the greedy "I can control this or that because I'm rich or because I have whatever job or because I'm an old white male or I'm an entitled middle age woman or I'm this or that CEO or a board president or blah blah blah." That is all from the ego. I mean the power we are born with. It is the power of knowing you are made out of the same stuff as the stars in the universe—the power in feeling the divine within your being. It is the power in finding peace in the chaos, light in the dark, joy in the sadness. *This* is true power. *This* is what you can control. Own it. Simply to breathe in and breathe out is such a treasure and helpful guide. Feel that breath? That is spirit moving in you. God is with you every second of the way.

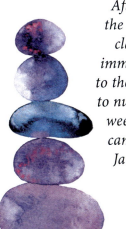

After finishing the Noque 12km classic race, I immediately went to the spectator bus to nurse an eleven-week-old Kate. I came in second. January 2017.

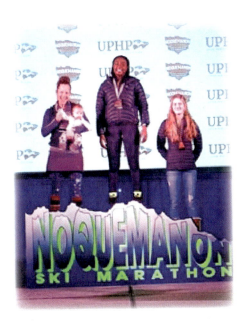

"My passion and fire run deep through my veins, my blood, there's no doubt about that."

— *Carolyn Aronson*

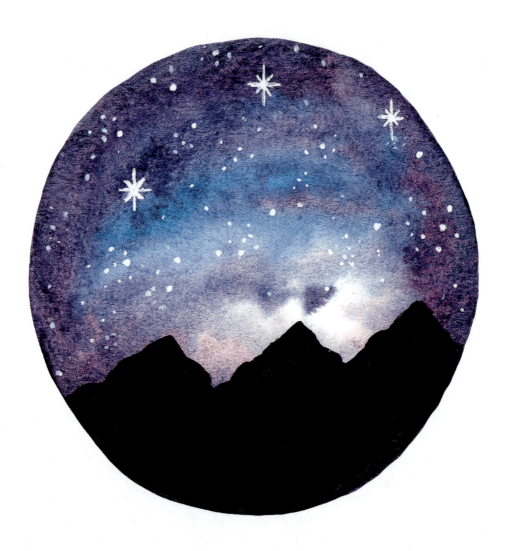

Chakra Guiding Questions

Solar Plexus Chakra

Close your eyes and bring your attention to your core, your power center, your solar plexus chakra. This is the energy center located in the core of your body that connects to your energy, will, personal power, and autonomy. When balanced, you feel flexible and at peace, protected, and comfortable with yourself and others. Check in with your body and mind. Do an honest gut check and ask yourself where you are.

Do you feel powerful? **YES**   No

What makes you feel powerful?

_____

_____

_____

If someone or something is making you feel powerless, what can *you* do to stop it?

_____

_____

_____

What can you do...what steps can you take...to regain some of your God-given power?

_____

_____

_____

What are you passionate about? What fuels your fire? What would you like to see more of?

_____

_____

_____

Chakra Training Tips
Solar Plexus (Fire) Chakra

Visualization: As you inhale and exhale, picture a ball of fire rising to the sun, stretching your core and spine up as well. Breathe in and lift. Breathe out and relax. Feel the energy radiate out and fill your whole body with warmth and light.

Positive Affirmations: I am enough. I accept myself. I stand confident in my power. I respect differences. I follow my passions. I am a changemaker.

Crystal Therapy: Topaz, citrine, yellow zircon, amber, tiger eye.

Nutrition: Yellow foods.

Aromatherapy: Grapefruit, ginger, lemongrass, blue tansy.

This chakra is connected to the element of fire. Burn incense, light a candle, or diffuse the suggested essential oils. Explore the many others; trust your instincts.

Sound Therapy: Chant *ram* in the key of E; listen to a roaring fire.

Yoga Poses: Bridge, boat, bow, half lord of the fishes.

Healing with Nature: Spend time with friends around a bonfire; sit in the full light of the sun.

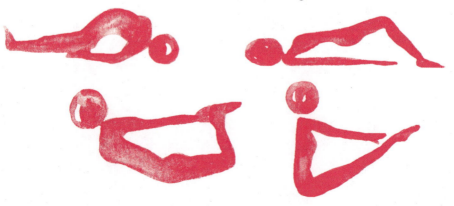

NOTES:

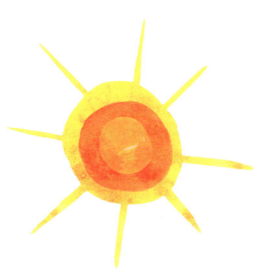

Be Extraordinary

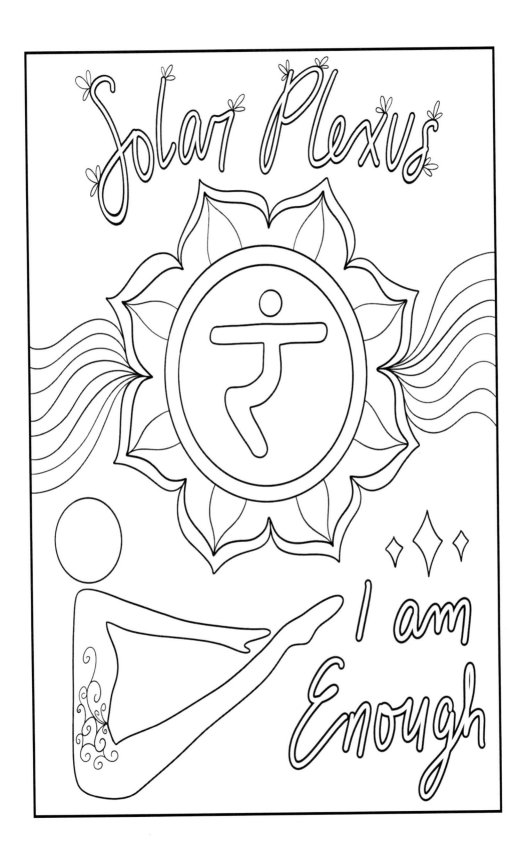

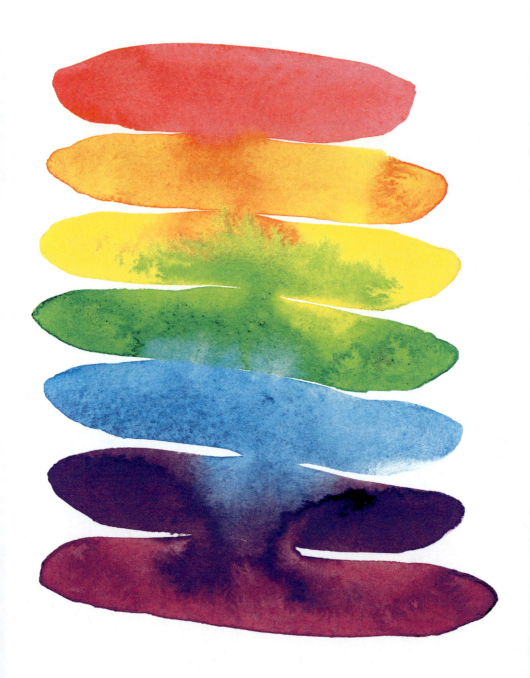

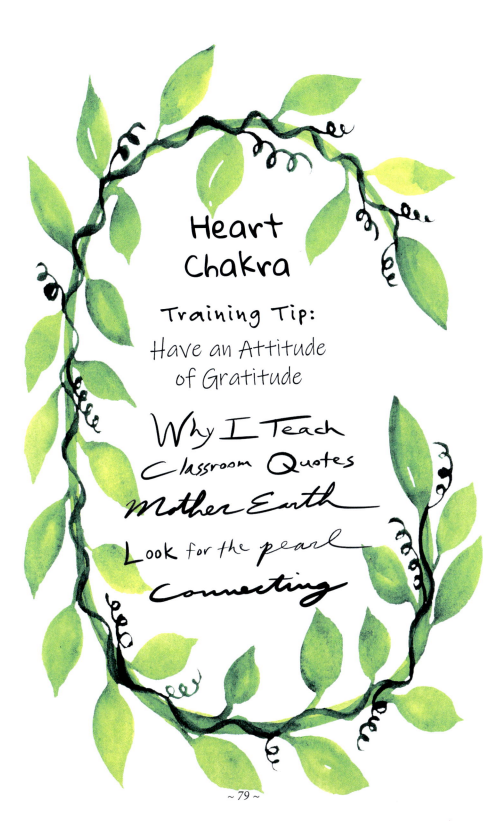

Heart Chakra

Training Tip:
Have an Attitude of Gratitude

Why I Teach

Classroom Quotes

Mother Earth

Look for the pearl

Connecting

You are loved.
You are love.
Everything
you need
is already
inside.

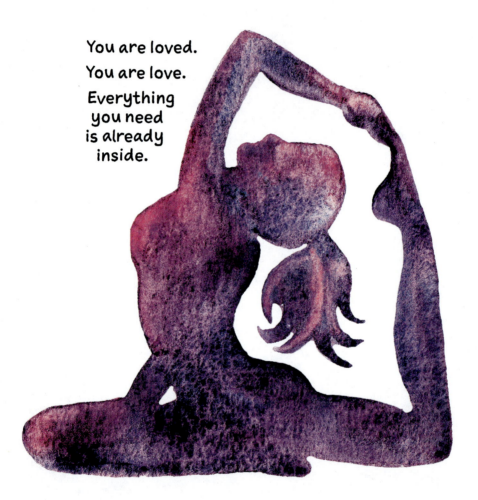

Why I Teach

My heart chakra has been super-energized my entire life. I care deeply. I feel everything. I basically wear my heart on my sleeve. It's who I am. I am grateful for everything—the good and the bad. You can't have one without the other. It's the yin and yang of life. There needs to be a balance. The not so good helps us appreciate the good. I'm grateful for my health and ability to run, bike, and ski to my heart's content. I'm grateful for our home and the tiny humans we're raising. I'm dearly grateful for my husband Erich. My family takes up a huge portion of my heart.

My job (which is more than just that) takes up another big chamber in my heart. The best teachers know that education is a calling. I was truly called to this field and basically feel I've been teaching my entire life, whether it was helping my younger brother growing up, guiding numerous kids I've babysat, or teaching little ones to ski, which I've done since middle school.

Teaching, like my love for silent sports, is also in my blood. My mom was an art teacher. Her mom was a chemistry and home economics teacher for a short time. Her dad was an agricultural science and welding teacher for forty-four years. My mom's grandpa was on the school board and used to ride around in his horse-drawn sleigh to pick up kids on

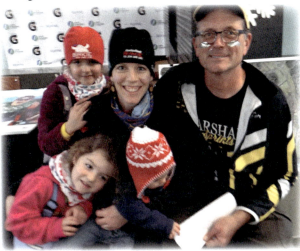

Emma, Hali, Kate, and me with the best coach ever, Dave Johnson. We drove four hours to an event at the new Grand Avenue Nordic Center in Duluth, Minnesota, for the opportunity to hear Jessie Diggins speak and to work out with an Olympic Gold Medalist. November 2018.

the farms in the middle of winter to take them to school. Their passion and dedication to teaching and learning and helping kids be successful ran deep. I am so grateful to have followed in their footsteps. I am honored to carry on that legacy.

I don't remember when I decided to go to school for teaching. Besides my family, I believe one very special person helped steer me in that direction, Dave Johnson. He was my high school ski coach and also a teacher. He brought me along as a nanny when he took his wife and two young children on a month-long adventure in England and Wales the summer before my senior year. It was an epic trip.

The advice he gave me when I was a nervous, impressionable sixth grader has stuck with me. He told me he had the best job in the world! He was always positive and knew exactly how to bring out the best in everyone. He still does. He had a profound effect on me, and I knew I wanted to be that person for others as well.

I ran and skied in college, but more importantly, I went to Gustavus to become a teacher. I received the best education from my professors and mentor teachers during my years in southern Minnesota. I graduated in 2006 and walked across the sweltering outdoor stage with a deep sense of pride. My first teaching job was right out of college in a kindergarten classroom at Lincoln Elementary in Saint Cloud, Minnesota. I'll never forget that class and those kids. Lucias and Moesha, Shannon, Duncan…I wonder where *"all ya'll are at"* these days. I wonder if you remember me. I wonder if you know what you meant to me. You will always be in my heart. I love you all and hope you're well.

Do you want to know my all-encompassing, effervescent, second-by-second, breath-by-breath prayer as an educator? To quote the great Albert Einstein, "Education is not the learning of facts, but the training of the mind to think." As educators, it is our deepest responsibility, our honor, and our great joy to teach children and young adults…

- ♥ To think of others.
- ♥ To think before they speak.
- ♥ To think of thoughtful resolutions to problems.
- ♥ To think of the best answer rather than the quickest.
- ♥ To think about their role in society and how they can make a difference.
- ♥ To think about their strengths rather than their weaknesses.
- ♥ To think with an open mind and open heart.
- ♥ To think with a positive attitude.
- ♥ To think about the implications of their actions.
- ♥ To think creatively.
- ♥ To think beyond the four walls of a classroom.
- ♥ To think mindfully and act boldly.
- ♥ To think responsibly.
- ♥ To think about how to serve people in need.
- ♥ To think about how to respectfully disagree.
- ♥ To think about the beauty of diversity.
- ♥ To think about tolerance and acceptance.
- ♥ To think about their dreams.
- ♥ To think about their limitless potential.
- ♥ To think about their similarities to others rather than their differences.
- ♥ To think about how to be agents of change and peddlers of peace.
- ♥ To think calmly and clearly during times of conflict.
- ♥ To think for themselves.

You will not find these things written on lesson plans. They can only be found by listening to a teacher's heartbeat. Herein lies the paradox. In a world of scantrons and standardized tests, students are not graded on these intangibles, teachers are not evaluated on them, schools are not rated on them. But these are the *exact* things we should all be held accountable for. Don't you agree?

I will continue to teach the way I do because I know it matters. It's in my heart. We need to use our spiritual gifts to do the most good we can, to lift others up, to build bridges, not walls. Amen? We are all connected. We are all members of the human race. We are all worthy of education, literacy, decency, and love! That's why I teach. To honor the children, to make a difference in countless lives, to influence the changemakers of tomorrow.

To all the teachers doing the important work of identifying white privilege and finding a more inclusive way, lifting up underrepresented, marginalized community members to allow their voices and stories to be heard, making it a point to have diversity and inclusion be the focal point of your teaching, having difficult conversations on important issues such as racism and other injustices, creating safe spaces for people to open up and share about their sexual orientation or their mental health or any other mountain they feel they're climbing, cultivating self-awareness and self-regulation strategies and teaching those in your circle to do the same, and not backing down when you are questioned.

You know who you are. You may feel like you're alone. You may feel scared to speak up. You may have been told to stay quiet. You may feel helpless at times. Please know this: You are not alone. You must be brave and speak up. Even if your voice shakes, you must. I believe in you. I'm right there with you doing the hard work. I know I'm speaking to the choir if you're still reading this, but it must be said; everyone deserves the right to pursue happiness. But if certain populations are not included in the conversation or the read alouds or the history being taught, that pursuit is near-impossible. It is our duty as humans to support one another no matter our differences, no matter our beliefs, no matter what. My heart goes out to all of you. Thank you for doing the important work wherever you are.

Children are brilliant beyond compare, overflowing with potential, filled with intuition and creativity, all of which can in no way be measured on a standardized test. The system is testing the curiosity, joy, and desire to keep learning and exploring right out of our children, and it needs to stop. And you know what else? Teachers are brilliant beyond compare, overflowing with generosity, talent, and wisdom. They go above and beyond, spend their own hard-earned money, and risk their lives for all our children. They deserve to be treated and paid like the heroic professionals they are. Can I get an amen?

I've taught early kindergarten, kindergarten, second grade, title one, sixth, seventh, and eighth grade language arts, and

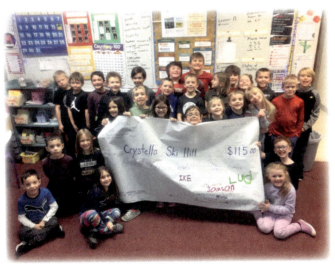

The second-grade class of 2019-2020…the year my time with these amazing human beings was cut short due to COVID 19. My incredible teaching partner Lauri Patterson and I led our students through a Michigan Project Place lesson on economics. The kids learned about local nonprofits and businesses. We toured a local business. They learned about so many economic concepts in a real-world manner. In the end, they raised $230 to donate to two great causes in the community.

high school language arts at an alternative education center. You know how I didn't teach them? With scantrons and yes or no questions. I didn't stand up there and lecture. All good teachers know these things don't work. I let kids explore, get messy, be problem **solvers**, readers, writers, and *thinkers*! I held poetry readings in local coffee shops, brought in inspirational and diverse speakers to share their culture, stood on desktops and sang, sat underneath desks and listened, shared my many journals to encourage growth, took them out in nature, and created community.

Classroom Quotes

I'd like to share with you just a few quotes and stories I've collected from my years as a teacher. Many of the wise words I have heard over the years have been lost in the chasm of my brain, but they have all made a significant difference in my heart and made me a better person. Maybe they will inspire you to go back to school to become a teacher. Maybe they'll whisper to you to encourage your own children or grandchildren to go into education. It is a noble field, indeed. Maybe they'll invite you to send a thank you note to an old teacher, your child's teacher, or the principal. Maybe you'll hear a whisper to teach

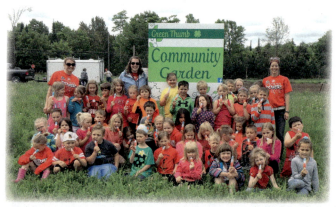

2016: Me with my colleagues, Jackie Giuliani and Lisa Cousineau. This was the year the school decided to get rid of Early Fives so the kindergarten class was huge. We walked half a block to the community garden to do some spring cleaning and prep work.

abroad and serve in a school far outside your comfort zone. Maybe you'll donate to a cause that's fighting for education for all (Save the Children, UNICEF, Room to Read, just to name a few). Maybe you'll feel compelled to write or call the people in power to tell them what you think truly matters in education. Maybe you are one of those people in power and you'll get the courage to speak up for the future of our children and make some changes in legislation to provide proper and equitable funding to our schools or to pass bills that support and protect all those you serve, especially the marginalized populations.

"I love it when you give me hugs."

"Mrs. Ziegler, you haven't hugged me in a while."

"You know what's special about the strawberry? The seeds are on the outside."

"I love you. I love how you teach us in so many different ways."

"You have the most beautiful eyes."

"Your eyes sparkle like the sun and moon."

Seriously, these kids have my heart. They could teach adults a thing or two about world peace! In the next election, I'm voting for Kid President for president. And not too long from now, I'll be voting for one of my own students! That's right, Owen Hendricks. Keep believing in yourself as much as I believe in you.

You know what else I encouraged? Using manners, giving compliments, always trying your best, and choosing to be kind. Every. Single. Day. Education is more than the required curriculum. Education is much more than the Common Core!

It's teaching...

common courtesy.

common sense.

common ground.

"Education is not the filling of a bucket but the lighting of a *fire*." And going back to the fire of our solar plexus, I also incorporated mindful movement and mindfulness every day. From intention setting and gratitude journaling to breathing exercises and appreciation circles and everything in between. Not required, but absolutely essential to the success and well-being of students (and teachers) everywhere. Giving them tools to cope with their big emotions and embodying those strategies myself allowed them to settle in, calm down, self-regulate, find solutions to problems, and learn to their greatest potential.

"You're the best teacher ever!"

"You're my most favorite teacher."

"I just love this classroom so much." (Picture a five-year-old sprawled on the floor trying to give it a hug.)

"I miss you every night."

"You are an angel."

"You make my heart happy."

On Martin Luther King, Jr. Day, I asked the kids to think about what their dreams were. One kid replied, "That you would be my mom."

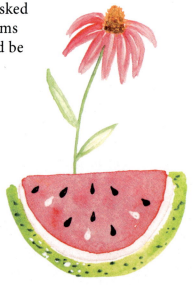

"Everybody in here is a good writer; they just have to find it in them."

— *Middle School Boy.*

(Seriously, I should've received an award for that comment.)

"Can I come back to your class? I miss you."

"You look like a flower."

"You look like a watermelon."

"Your room is like heaven on earth."

Now there's a comparison I never thought I'd hear to describe my classroom. How can I top that? Wow. That was by far the best, most extraordinary compliment I've received in all my years of teaching. With a close second being, "You're just like Miss Frizzle." And a close third being, "You're a hero."

I also taught my students about climate change, even my kindergarteners. From the science behind what the problem is, to working through their feelings and frustrations, to guiding them to simple solutions. Here's why: Children influence their parents and other grownups in their circle. These adults will then be nudged a little at a time to continue the conversation, to analyze their own way of living and personal carbon footprint, and to make changes. It matters.

It's our deep responsibility as educators (and adults) to show children the facts, show them how their daily choices affect the earth and the climate and what can be done. I taught them about climate change to encourage them to change their habits (and again influence their parents). In a society that's all about consume, consume, consume, stuff, stuff, stuff, new, new, new, deal, deal, deal, our brains have been trained to do just that. We simply don't need more plastic garbage in our homes…even if it's only $2—unless we want a world like the one created by the brilliant minds behind the movie *WALL-E*. Let's not let that happen. As a teacher, my job is to retrain their brains.

These next few quotes came from me during the two years I taught middle school language arts. While I never envisioned myself teaching sixth, seventh, and eighth graders, I did it to help the district, and I *loved* getting them to write more. I was dealing with my second miscarriage the first year I taught middle school and our first born and maternity leave the second year. These were just a couple of the extenuating circumstances that made teaching hormonal pre-teens that much more…interesting.

"The seven minutes have begun. I feel like these seven minutes are more like seven hours for this group. Holy wah! Boy can this group drive me nuts. Good thing we're running intervals at practice today. I need to blow off steam, big time. Okay, Chandra, look for the pearl…most of them are writing, writing, writing. Focus on them. Find the good. Breathe in. Breathe out. All is well."

"This year has been more of a challenge than a pleasure. Maybe I'll look back and realize this group made me a better teacher, but honestly, I don't want to look back. I need to look forward."

Here's the truth. Teaching is *hard*! I had many periods of self-doubt, feeling like a failure—stressed, anxiety-ridden, and totally frustrated. There were a few times I wanted to quit. I thought I could be a better mother if I weren't completely emotionally drained at the end of every day. Physically, many days I felt like I had run a marathon. Teaching takes a lot of heart and extraordinary endurance, especially if you want to stay in it for the long haul. It has to be for the kids, always for the kids. They are my why. The relationships. The chance to make a difference in so many lives. The opportunity to inspire greatness. Teachers don't go into education for the money, that's for sure. But I wouldn't complain if a person in power decided to pay us like educators in Finland. Or simply give us the resources needed to teach safely during a global pandemic.

Mother Earth

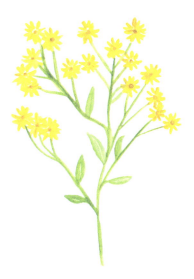

You know what else takes a lot of endurance—*living*. Sometimes, the simplest acts of living are the hardest to endure. Trying to survive when life throws us shit and finding a way to wade through it all and *thrive* takes real endurance.

Dear Reader, I know we all have such beautifully diverse backgrounds and experiences, which I guess is another reason I want to write books. I want to reach multiple audiences, bridge gaps, and make connections. I want to show that we are more alike than we are different. Imagining all the different people reading this at the same time fills me with joy and makes my heart chakra overflow.

One thing I am eternally grateful for is what we all have in common—the ground we walk on, the place we all call home, our planet earth, our Mother Earth. *She* has the most endurance of all. We could learn a lot from her. Nature is truly the best teacher.

I love nature dearly. *She* needs *all* of us to come together and put her back together. She needs our collective knowledge, gifts, and wisdom to stop climate change and to help her heal and restore life, love, peace, and balance. She is powerful, patient, precious, and priceless. We cannot tread on her so heavily anymore. We must right our wrongs and make a conscious effort to love *her* more—and as a result, love ourselves and each other more. Can I get an amen for Mother Earth? Ultimately, she will be okay. She can endure almost anything. What we need to start thinking about is how we can live in greater harmony with her or *we* will be the ones not okay (as in, *we* will go extinct).

If you are grateful for the air you breathe, the water you drink, the land you call home and upon which you can enjoy silent sports, if you give thanks for your freedom and your food, then please, show your gratitude in actions and not just words. Walk or bike more. Carpool. Travel less. Purchase carbon offsets. Shop locally. Buy used. Buy less. Recycle. Compost your food scraps. Start your own garden. Switch to LED bulbs. Turn things off and unplug them when not in use. Sign up for renewable energy (if possible). Turn your heat up or down a degree or two. Use water wisely. Have healthy conversations about climate change. Talk to local elected officials about

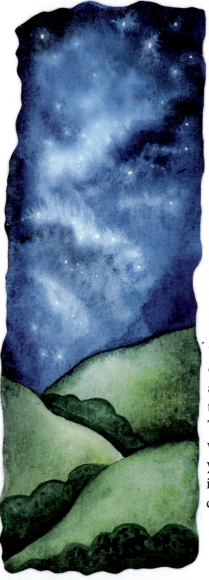

green policies. Write or call state and national legislators and ask for them to take action. Read the book, *Climate Change: Musings and Stories from Lake Superior's North Shore* by Katya Gordon. It's an easy read with stories about how climate change is affecting everyone, even the people from her small town, Two Harbors, Minnesota.

The Higher Power you believe in will thank you for your concerted efforts. It's okay if you don't believe. The Great Spirit believes in you and thanks you anyway. You know who else will thank you? Your grandchildren. When they ask you someday what you did to help stop the global pandemic of climate change (and COVID 19), you'll be able to look them in the eye and tell them honestly that you did your part. Think of them. Also, think of them when you make decisions about how you choose to live. You will have incredible stories to share from our collective time in quarantine.

We need a revolution
And it starts with you
When you heal yourself
You heal the universe
When you take time for yourself
You take time for the universe
When you are kind to yourself
You are kind to the universe
When you love yourself
You love the universe
For, you see, you are the universe
Held to the same cosmic laws of
the universe
Made of the same particles as
all the shining stars in our ever-
expanding miraculous universe
Let your inner light shine
You were born to shine
Know that we are cosmically and
intimately connected
Recognize that when you take care
of yourself, your whole being is
filled with positive healing energy,
and that energy radiates into the
universe
Peace
Love
Harmony
Unity
Hope
Tolerance
Kindness
It's possible
Because you are possible
Our world needs a revolution
And it starts with you

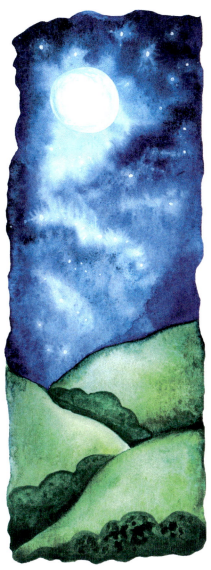

Look for the Pearl

As a teacher, a mom, and a human being, I've always insisted on having an attitude of gratitude. We need to be grateful for what we've got. We need to give thanks for our gifts, for wild places, and for all life. We need to act upon our heartfelt gratitude. We need to look for the pearl.

I believe it was my kindergarten methods teacher, Mary O'Brien, who introduced me to this mantra. Thank you, Mary. I'm grateful for the things you taught me. To look for the pearl simply means to find the good in a situation or person. There will be plenty of darkness, but we need to intentionally seek the light—to be on the lookout for all that is good in our lives.

Even when I was down in the pits after breaking my collarbone in 2018, I was grateful. I was grateful for my husband Erich who loved me so much, who believed in me when I didn't believe in myself, who washed my hair and helped me get dressed, who endured my tears, who did everything around the house. I was grateful for my daughters' words. "Are you okay, Mom?" and "I'll help you heal." I was grateful for good friends and colleagues who brought dinner for us. I was grateful for the helmet on my head that protected my brain when I went over my handlebars. I was grateful for so much because I knew in the whole scheme of things, I was fine, and *we* were doing just fine. I knew my condition was only temporary, and I'd be back in my running shoes in no time.

My heart is so open that sometimes I take on too much of other people's stuff. Who can relate? Again, we're all works in progress. We can be compassionate, empathetic, helpful, and loving, yet remain stable and calm at the same time. We must first balance our lower chakras. We must bring awareness to the strength, energy, and true power of our thoughts and emotions. We must find a way to dive deeply within ourselves.

Imagine yourself in the midst of a torrential rain in the middle of the ocean. On the surface, everything appears dark, scary, and out of control. Yet if you dive beneath the surface, you'll find calm water, peace, and serenity. The same can be applied to many situations that tug at our hearts and make us feel such strong emotions.

So, we must dive deep into the crevasses of our hearts where pure love and complete calmness reside. I'm not here to tell you it's easy. I struggle with this. I have three daughters! They are full of passion and fire and drama and energy to the max. They love each other fiercely and can fight with the best of them.

Trust me, I don't always dive deeply into my happy place. Once I even left in the middle of the girls fighting without telling anyone. I needed to let off some steam before I could find that serenity. I ran down our ski trail into the woods. I huffed and puffed and screamed up to the sky. And then...all was calm. Or at least I felt more in control and returned home to deal with the situation.

Also, I simply do what I love and live authentically. I do what makes me happy 90 percent of the time. Life has its must dos that aren't exactly happiness-inducing but must be done, nevertheless. Things happen to us or our loved ones that are not at all happy. Then there are things we wish we could do more of that we're sure would bring us great joy (traveling) but we don't. Aim for 90 percent.

But here's the thing: Those are all external stimuli that... You. Cannot. Control. What you *can* control is the way you respond, your attitude. You choose what to focus on in any given situation. If you choose the good (the pearl), you will attract more good. If you choose to focus on the bad and just dwell in that tide pool that isn't going anywhere, then chances are pretty good you will go nowhere.

If you're a little skeptical about that, that's okay. That's where you are. But also, let me be the first to tell you your skepticism is exactly what's keeping you from living your happiest life and fulfilling all the dreams in your heart. Life is too short. Let yourself be happy. Let yourself be free—free from comparison, free from too many commitments, free from constant attachment to technology, free from disease, free from anything else stopping you.

Mother Nature (or God) threw us *all* a curve ball when she sent us to our rooms for a long timeout during the COVID-19 global pandemic. She wanted us to think long and hard about our choices and how we were treating her and our brothers and sisters. She wanted us to *free* ourselves from all those things mentioned above. She wanted us to slow down and spend more time connecting with her and our loved ones. She wanted us to think about how we can lighten the load upon our own lives while at the same time lightening the load we place upon her as well.

Letting myself be happy means having a clear conscience when it comes to my effect on the earth (asking myself, am I doing enough to lower my carbon footprint?) while filling my life with what I truly love. That means dancing and reading with my kids, giving lots of hugs and kisses, snuggling with my black labs, writing, painting, doing yoga, running, skiing, biking, camping, collecting rocks, lighting sage once in a while to clear the energy, reading about spirit animals and inspiring people (like Greta Thunberg, Malala, Jessie Diggins, the Nigerian school girls who were captured by Boko Haram, and more), shopping at St. Vinny's, Goodwill, and consignment stores, drinking good coffee, enjoying a glass of wine, not eating dairy, only eating meat that we've harvested ourselves or the meat from other like-minded people, recycling everything possible, listening to great music, not getting caught in a negative mindset when I read about all the crap going on in the world but rather reframing my thoughts to "What can I do?" and being the change I wish to see in the world.

Like I said before, I could go on and on. My heart is *so* full and open. I sometimes have to get away from it all. I need to retreat into my own shell to feel balanced and restored. (I am a true Cancer.) And I think that's okay. You are invited to take a timeout. You are invited to retreat to wherever possible—a cave in the hills of Tibet is not really possible most of the time, but a quiet lake, the woods, a retreat of any kind, the library, your bedroom, the bathroom, even your car will do. Take a timeout from it all. Disconnect to reconnect. Reconnect with your mind, body, and spirit. You are three in one. Take care of *all* of you. *Love* all that you are. Give thanks for where you've been, where you are, and where you're going. Mostly, give thanks for the present.

Connecting

Here are other ways I connect with my heart chakra to bring emotional healing:

- I cry.

- I get angry...ugly angry sometimes...then cry some more, and eventually wring my heart free from the constrictor grip of anger, the source of which is evolutionary at its core. My dear friend Amanda Rasner opened my mind to the concept of righteous anger. She said, "I believe anger over injustice is a justified anger that moves us to compassion and action." It made total sense to me. There are many sources and reasons to be angry from the mistreatment of our earth to the mistreatment of people of color, the LGBTQ+ community, women, children, and immigrants. It is okay to have these strong feelings. It's what makes us uniquely human. It's what compels us to be the change we wish to see.

- But you know what, I also cry over everyday frustrations sometimes. It's easy to get caught in this cycle. I let it out; then I move on. I know I need to raise my frequency and radiate positivity.

- I forgive others. I believe everyone is doing the best they can. I accept that what was done came from their current level of consciousness. I know they are on their own path of spiritual evolution toward forgiveness and enlightenment.

- I forgive myself.

- I am completely open.

"If future generations are to remember us more with gratitude than sorrow,

we must achieve more than just the miracles of technology.

We must also leave them a glimpse of the world as it was created,

not just as it looked when we got through with it."

— *Lyndon B. Johnson*

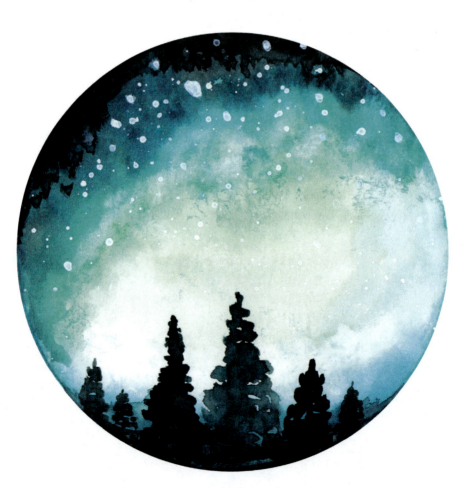

Chakra Guiding Questions

Heart Chakra

Close your eyes and focus on your heart chakra. Feel into the energy pulsing from this area of your physical body. This is the energy center located in the region of your heart that connects you to your emotional self. When balanced, you feel joy, love, gratitude, compassion, and forgiveness. Listen. What is it saying? How does it feel?

Do you love yourself?

_____

_____

_____

How could you love yourself more?

_____

_____

_____

What makes your heart the happiest?

_____

_____

_____

What do you want to manifest?

_____

_____

_____

How are you loving others and *all* living things?

_____

_____

_____

How can you change to be more loving and compassionate?

_____

_____

_____

In what ways do you or can you express gratitude?

_____

_____

_____

NOTES:

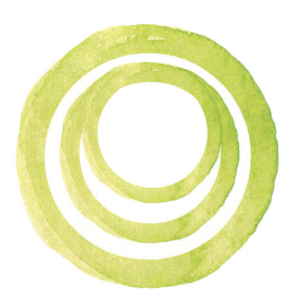

Chakra Training Tips

Heart (Air) Chakra

Visualization: As you inhale and exhale, picture a green rosebud at the center of your chest, slowly unfolding. Breathe in and imagine the bud opening. Breathe out and let go of what no longer serves you. Be patient as you steady your breath and feel yourself bloom.

Positive Affirmations: I love myself. I love others. I am grateful for all the blessings in my life. I release all my fears and concerns. I am one.

Crystal Therapy: Malachite, jade, green tourmaline, emerald, chrysoprase, peridot.

Nutrition: Green foods.

Aromatherapy: Ylang ylang, rose, bergamot.

This chakra is connected to the element of air so simply breathe in the aromas of pure therapeutic-grade essential oils and feel love and compassion fill every cell of your physical body.

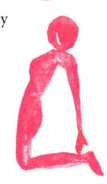

Sound Therapy: Chant *yam* in the key of F, listen to wind.

Yoga Poses: Forward bend, camel, cat, cobra.

Healing with Nature: Connect to the wind, practice deep breathing, and any kind of cardio such as walking, running, biking, snowshoeing, or skiing.

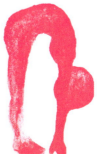

Be Extraordinary

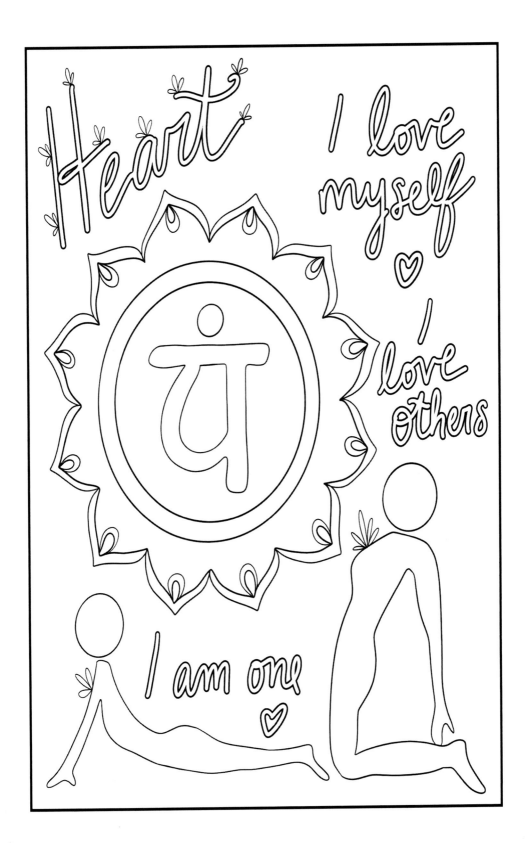

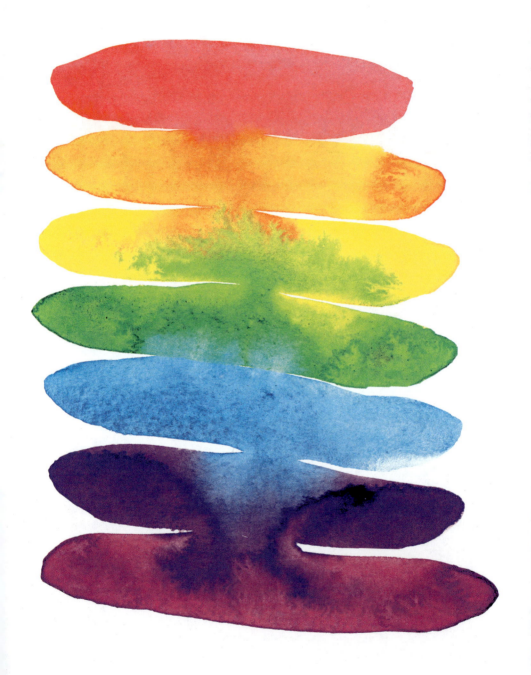

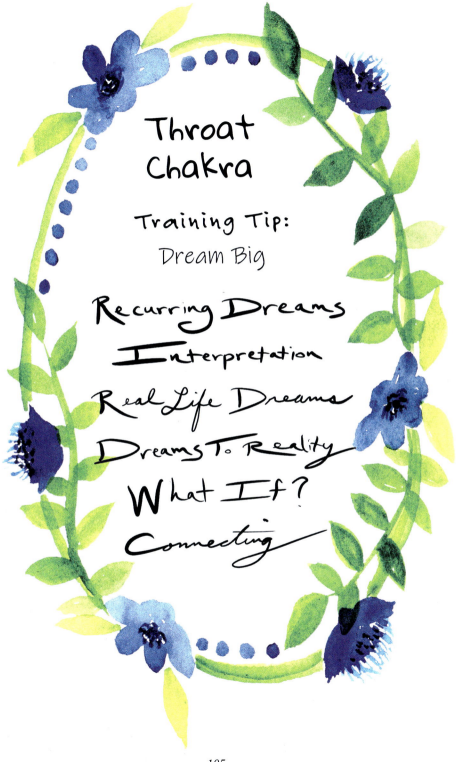

Throat Chakra

Training Tip:
Dream Big

Recurring Dreams

Interpretation

Real Life Dreams

Dreams To Reality

What If?

Connecting

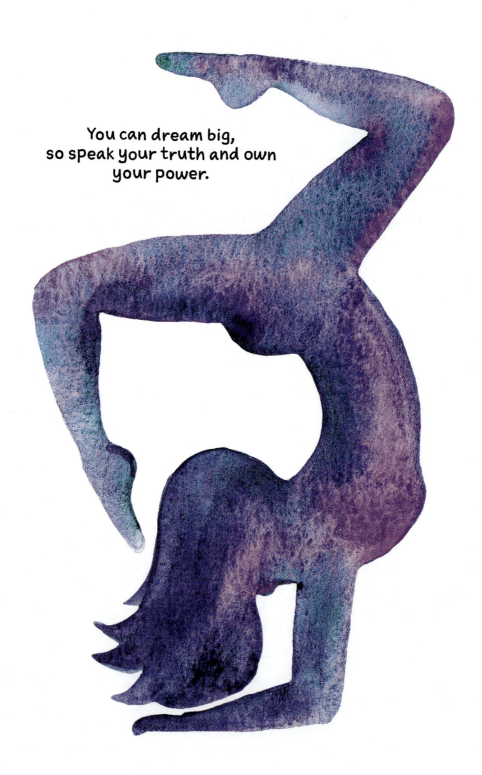

You can dream big,
so speak your truth and own
your power.

Recurring Dreams

Over the years, I've had two major recurring dreams. One is of me running a race, but I'm either running painfully in slow motion or I'm not dressed to run and I'm wearing a backpack. The other has been happening more recently. It's of me running a race, but it turns into a maze of sorts, going in and out of buildings, different doors, and tight spaces. In both dreams, I feel incredibly helpless, frustrated, and frankly, pissed off. In both dreams, I never finish the race.

I've tried willing my legs to move faster, but they won't. I've tried going back to the same dream to go the "right" way, but I can't. I've asked myself time and time again what these dreams are trying to tell me.

The obvious answer is that something or someone is slowing me down. Or could it be, according to dream interpretation expert Anna-Karin Bjorklund, "Unforeseen obstacles in dreams can represent external changes happening in your life which you might not be fully comfortable with."

Then I started going to this class called Energetically Simple in my tiny town led by a delightfully enlightened lady named Barbara Luck. I found out some time later that we have the same birthday, twenty years apart. No wonder I felt a soul-sister connection with her and felt at home immediately. I just wanted more and more of the energy, the shifts in my soul, the rise in my spirit, the perfectly impeccable miraculous timing of everything, the feeling that I was living life in full color, growing and evolving with an amazing tribe of wise and wonderful women.

During the third or fourth class, I mentioned my recurring dreams. Barb might know my soul, but she didn't know I had been running and skiing practically my whole life and that endurance athletes cannot sit still (unless it's a rest day). Here's a summary of her interpretation of my dreams, "You need to slow down." I thought, *Are you serious? Slow down?*

Then, like a flash, I was reminded of my mountain bike crash that had happened about three months earlier.

Interpretation

My new friend Barb said my dreams were telling me I needed to slow down. Also, apparently, when you can't figure out what your dreams are trying to tell you, the Universe sends another sign. Unfortunately (or fortunately, depending on your frame of thinking), my sign was a major kick in the ass right over my handlebars and onto my face, breaking me to pieces and forcing me to stop *all* movement! Message received.

During my first run post-collarbone surgery, which I mentioned earlier, as with most of my runs, I remained silent, not distracted by music in my ears. I listened to the music of the woods. The whispers in the wind. I also asked myself (my spirit guides, animals, God, the Universe) many, many questions. Where exactly are you leading me? Am I on the right path? What more should I be doing? Which of my dreams should I be following? Where are we going? I wish I had a clear answer.

I receive whispers and nudges now and then. I have learned to pay attention to my intuition (and to the signs of the Universe). I have learned that things happen for a reason and in their own time. I have learned to surrender to God's plans. But I have also learned that sometimes you just need to *be* the change. We're living a free will experiment and can't just sit around waiting for a dove or the sea to part.

So, what do I do about those nudges and signs? Do I truly need to slow down even more than I have? I honestly think I do slow down (when I can). I kept a gratitude journal every day for an entire *year, twice* (in both 2017 and 2020). That's slowing down and another book in itself. And really, I wake up in gratitude and go to sleep in gratitude as well. I sit and snuggle and read with my daughters every chance I get. I pet my black labs and feel really, truly happy. I go to an awesome church and slow down through song, prayer, and conversation. I teach a yoga class and go to a spirituality class where we sit and breathe.

I close my eyes, ground myself, and intentionally soak up every ounce of these moments because I know and believe with all my heart what a blessing each of those things is.

On the flip side, even after the crash, I feel like I can't slow down with everything going on in my life. How can I possibly slow down when I'm passionate about so many things? When there is so much to learn and discover? When there are so many injustices all around the world and I wish I could help or solve them all? I feel like Alexander Hamilton with a million things I have not done.

This truly is where I need the most guidance. I take on so much because I care, but I often end up feeling like a human doing rather than a human being.

Help me out, Universe. Where and how exactly do you want me to slow down? Where are you leading me? Please send me some signs. I'm all ears, eyes, everything. Just please don't send me over the handlebars again.

Just a few months after writing this section, we were sent the coronavirus. I guess my dreams were a collective dream of humanity. We all needed to slow down, eh? We all needed time to sit in silence and reflect on what truly mattered. We all needed more time and space to listen to our own nudges and to be present for ourselves and our families.

Real Life Dreams

So, what about the dreams I have for myself in real life? I have a lot of dreams, from being the best mom possible and raising girls who love and serve God and others with all their heart and soul, to traveling the world, to spending time with elephants, to running the Boston Marathon, to opening a yoga studio. I dream that the children I teach, the words I speak, and the books I write will affect so much positive change that the peace and harmony in the world will far outweigh the destruction. I dream of a world that no longer relies on fossil fuels to power cars, homes, and businesses. I dream of a world where every single human respects their worth and doesn't take themselves too seriously, lives by the golden rule, and respects the incredibly beautiful, diverse planet we all share. I dream of a world where everyone thinks critically and consumes consciously.

I also dream of my personal library being organized in rainbow order on bookshelves that line the walls of my house with a sliding ladder like Belle has in *Beauty and the Beast*. And I dream of converting an old school bus into a meditation retreat on wheels that I'll name Pearl. It will have a relaxation area in the back with cushions, glow-in-the-dark stars, and a diffuser with the perfect blend of oils to fit your needs. It will have shelves of books, a mini-kitchen to cook delicious nutritious meals, space to do some yoga, comfy places to sit and write, inspirational art, and wise words everywhere. It'll have everything you need to feed your body, mind, and soul. I will drive it around wherever I go and constantly remind people to "look for the pearl." If you can't find a pearl, I'll invite you aboard my bus and let you find one yourself. ☺ Oh, and of course, I'll have my rock collection along for the ride, and I'll invite you to decorate one with a word or phrase that will become your mantra. Everyone will be welcome. Doesn't that sound amazing?

Why do I have so many dreams that involve other people? I don't know. I guess life is more interesting and meaningful when we connect with others. What's it all for if we don't share kindness and spread light?

I also dream of just sitting on a beach somewhere all by myself. Soaking up the sun and the sound of the waves for as long as I want, then taking a leisurely stroll back home… wherever that may be, to hold hands with Erich, the love of my life.

Dreams to Reality

Do you know how to make your dreams come true? You think about them, write about them, *talk* about them, and then you take action. It starts with dreaming big and believing that you *can* and *will* accomplish whatever you set out to do. Write about your dreams often. I'm not talking about in a crazy, obsessive, this is all I can think about, life won't be good until I make these happen kind of way, but rather in a matter of fact, here are my dreams and I'm telling you, Universe, loud and clear that these will happen someday.

Making your dreams come true involves speaking your truth. You truly can think and speak your dreams into reality. Your thoughts will manifest in crazy, ridiculous ways. But also know that if you have a dream of running the Boston Marathon, you can't manifest your way into that one. You have to choose to do the work. You have to believe in your ability. You have to wake up early and lace up your shoes. Most dreams require physical action on your part, but I truly believe they all begin with thinking and speaking your truth.

Manifesting your dreams involves surrounding yourself with images and words of the exact things or feelings you want to achieve. Maybe that includes a vision board you do once a year. I've made a few of these, and I always enjoy the process. However, I'm the type of person who needs reminders everywhere. I have inspirational words and pictures on the kitchen cabinets, on the fridge, on a mirror in the basement, in my creation zone, in journals in every corner of the house, in my coat pockets, on my phone, everywhere.

Manifesting your dreams involves being brave and telling others. You will be pleasantly surprised by how beautifully things will begin to unfold, how people will offer guidance, and how often your dreams will come true. When I had the dream of being the first from my college to compete at the NCAA skiing championships, I started by telling myself that I could do it. Then I wrote it down. "I will make it to NCAAs." Then I told a few people—my coach, Erich, my sister. Then I did the work. I put in the blood, sweat, and tears for years, all while visualizing myself exactly where I wanted to be. When I was selected for the team, I was overjoyed, but I was not surprised. I knew I would get there. I believed in myself and worked incredibly hard.

Dreams do come true.

When I had the dream to write a book, again, it started with ideas in my head. Then I wrote it down in journals and on my phone. Then I told a few people. Then I shared the seedling of my story at a writing retreat. Then, as you already guessed, I did the work. I wrote and wrote, and I read and read, and I visualized myself holding the finished product. I eventually told more people and got the courage to send it to some publishing companies. And then, voilà!

When I had the dream to open a wellness center, well, that one's still a work in progress. If it's meant to be, I know the steps to making it happen. And anyway, I think you get my point.

Whatever your dream is, think about it. Start there. When the time feels good enough (because there is no such thing as the right time), write about it. Then talk about it. If you're only comfortable telling your pets, do that. You can also speak your ideas out loud to the trees or the stars or to your own reflection. Then, you need to act. Do one small thing every day to get closer to achieving your dream. And never stop believing in yourself.

What If?

What if you don't know how to dream or you forgot somewhere along the way? I hear you. Know that whatever you dream of is in your nature. Every child dreams *big* dreams. They also dream during the day as they play pretend and act on their "dreams" to create and sing and dance. It comes easily to them. Somewhere along the way, we lose that. We forget how to dream and play and think about our futures with rose-colored glasses (some never lose that).

We get overrun with all the requirements of adulthood. We read too much news. We busy ourselves with the daily grind and lose sight of the stars. We fail to notice the miraculous flower growing out of a crack in the sidewalk. We forget to look up. We falsely claim that we don't have time to (fill in the blank).

It's time to reclaim the magic of our youth. It's time to return to our inner truths and allow ourselves to dream both big and small.

To those asking, "What's the point?" I invite you to begin with visualizing. Start with the visualizations I provide after each section of this book, then branch out. While you're calm and relaxed and inviting good vibrations into your aura, put your dreams out there—no matter how crazy or absurd or sad or unrealistic they seem, do it *now*.

I mean right now!

Put this book down and just do it. No matter how weird it seems or where you are. Take your time. Put your bookmark in and come back when you're ready.

Welcome back. How'd you do? Doesn't it feel good?

Build on that start. Dream when your head is on your pillow before you go to sleep. Dream when your head is on your pillow before you get out of bed the next morning. Dream as you give thanks and sit in a moment of silence before you eat. Start small. Then build. Soon you'll be a dreaming machine, creating positive change in the world simply due to the higher energetic frequency you're putting out there. Amen?

You Are Allowed

You are allowed to dream big dreams.
You are allowed not to have any dreams.
You are allowed to try new things and make mistakes.
You are allowed to be brave and bold and reserved and timid at the same time.
You are allowed to wear dresses and running shorts.
You are allowed to like rock-'n'-roll and dance like a ballerina.
You are allowed to play pretend for as long as your heart desires.
You are allowed to do whatever makes you happy and break the mold.
You are allowed to cry and yell and scream and get angry at the world and the coronavirus.

You are allowed to feel all the feels and not feel in control.
You are allowed to smile even though you're sad about all the
human suffering.
You are allowed to be a light and spread joy endlessly.
You are allowed to let your light flicker in moments of despair
and let others do the heavy lifting.
You are allowed.

Chandra Ziegler
May 20, 2020

Connecting

Here are other ways I speak my truths and connect to my throat chakra:

- Between myself, God, my journals, my husband, my mom, my sister, my BRF (best running friend), my teaching partners, and my energy friends, I share everything that's on my mind and heart. I no longer hold anything in.

- I have healthy conversations with people about climate change.

- I march.

- I write to my elected officials and other people in power about issues that speak to my heart.

- I speak up at meetings when necessary.

- I have an open classroom where we can discuss difficult issues in a safe way.

- I write.

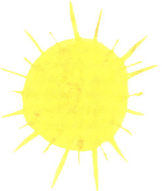

Marching and speaking at an Earth Day March for Science event in 2016 with my husband Erich, Emma, and Hali. I was pregnant with Kate. I'm sure she could feel my passion and fire for justice for all deep in the womb.

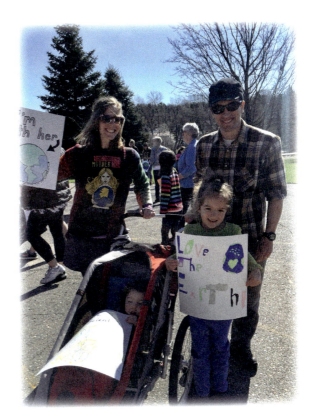

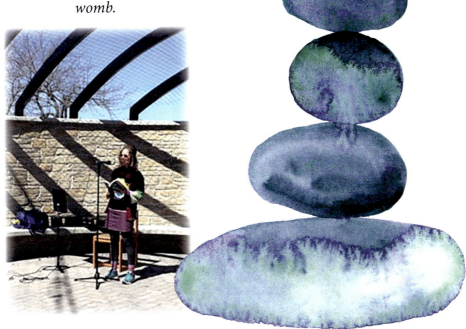

"We all have dreams.

But in order to make dreams come into reality,

it takes an awful lot of determination, dedication, self-discipline, and effort."

— *Jesse Owens*

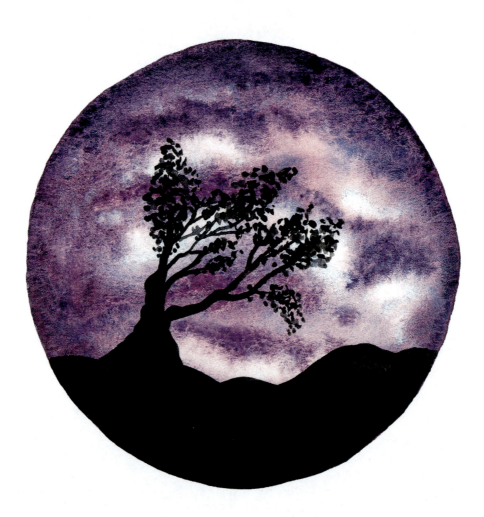

Chakra Guiding Questions

Throat Chakra

Close your eyes and bring your attention to your throat. How does it feel? Open? Constricted? Are there things you're holding back or not speaking?

Have you had any recurring dreams? What do you think they're trying to tell you?

_____

_____

_____

What dreams are in your heart?

_____

_____

_____

Have you ever told anyone your dreams?

_____

_____

_____

Who do you trust to share your dreams with?

_____

_____

_____

What small steps can you take today toward achieving your dreams?

_____

_____

_____

What haven't you told anyone but *really* need to get off your chest? Start by writing it down. If it feels right, tell someone. Do all things with love and kindness, and it'll be all right.

_____

_____

_____

How will you live life speaking your truths?

_____

_____

_____

NOTES:

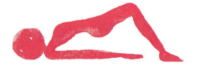

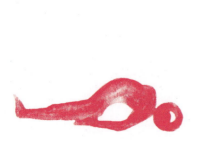

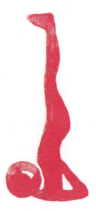

Chakra Training Tips

Throat Chakra

Visualization: As you inhale and exhale, picture something you love to eat against the blue sky. Breathe in and imagine tasting it as you also take in pure turquoise light. Breathe out and release any blockages in your throat. Continue this process until you feel confident to speak your mind.

Positive Affirmations: I speak my thoughts clearly with grace and integrity. I am aligned with my highest truth. I express who I am. I acknowledge the power of my words to shape my reality.

Crystal Therapy: Turquoise, blue agate, blue topaz, sapphire, aquamarine.

Nutrition: Fruits, juice, sauces, sea plants, soups, teas.

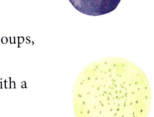

Aromatherapy: Spearmint, cassia (dilute with a carrier oil), lavender, basil.

Roll on pulse points or inhale.

Sound Therapy: Chant *ham* in the key of G; listen to sounds of birds or crickets.

Yoga Poses: Shoulder stand, plow, fish, bridge.

Healing with Nature: Take a walk outdoors on a sunny day.

Other: Sing your favorite songs, call a friend, write a letter.

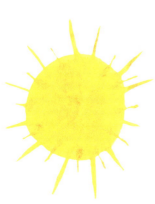

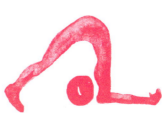

Be Extraordinary

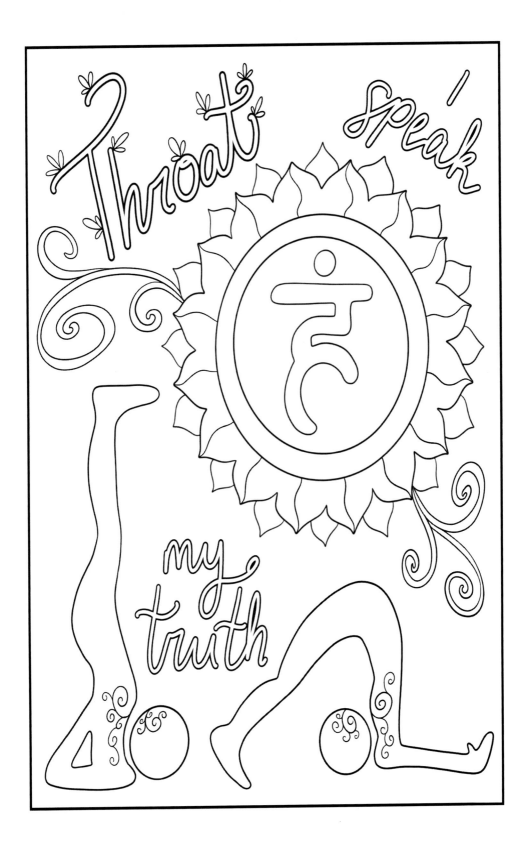

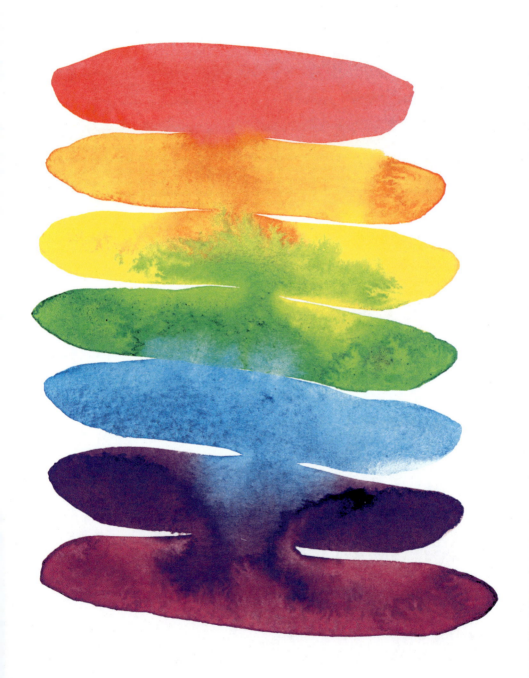

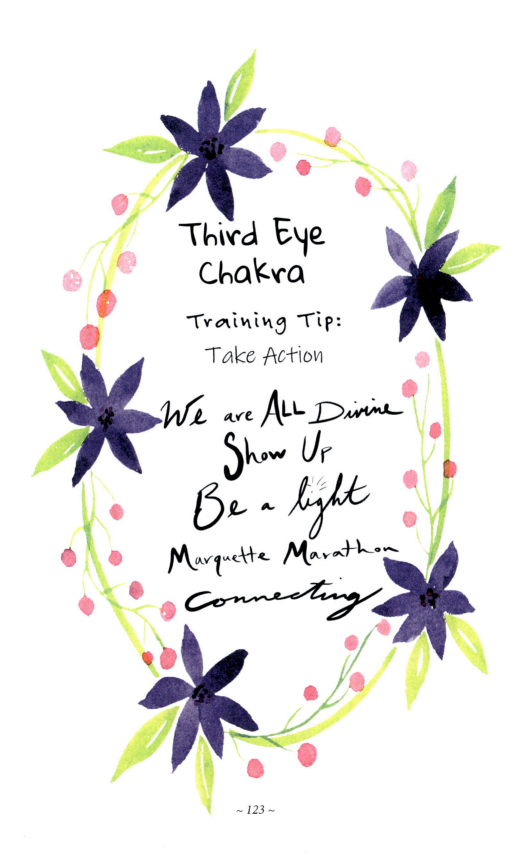

Third Eye Chakra

Training Tip:
Take Action

We are ALL Divine
Show Up
Be a light
Marquette Marathon
Connecting

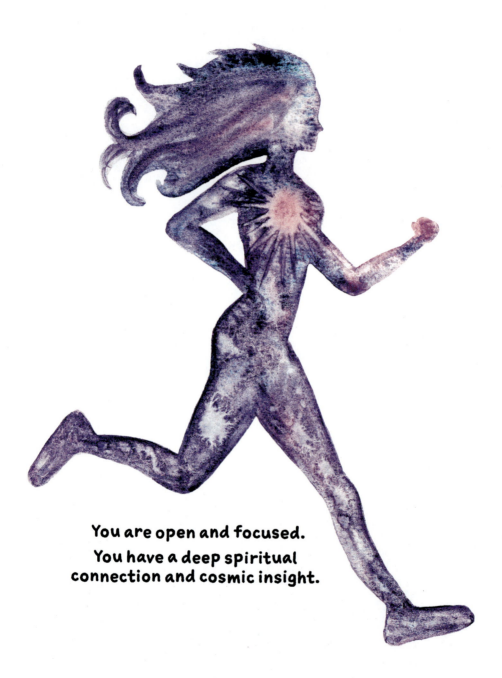

You are open and focused.
You have a deep spiritual
connection and cosmic insight.

We Are All Divine

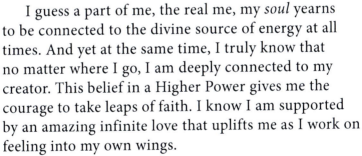

One night when I was in my thirties, I had yet another dream in which I unquestionably, unabashedly volunteered myself when a magician asked, "Who wants to learn how to fly?" I knew I was born to fly, to follow all my dreams and just soar. In the dream, I came so close. I was actually tethered together with a bunch of other people. I was standing at the edge of a tall building and was ready to make the leap. However, my dreams took me elsewhere or I woke up. I don't remember exactly. Either way, I didn't fly. I woke up and told myself, "You know what? No more holding back. I want to fly, dammit!"

Sometimes, I feel like an angel inside this body who does so much flying in my sleep, and then I wake up and I'm back on the ground again. I just want to keep flying—to follow all my dreams, to help fight injustice, to be free.

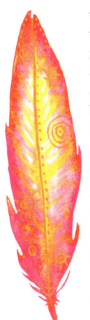

I guess a part of me, the real me, my *soul* yearns to be connected to the divine source of energy at all times. And yet at the same time, I truly know that no matter where I go, I am deeply connected to my creator. This belief in a Higher Power gives me the courage to take leaps of faith. I know I am supported by an amazing infinite love that uplifts me as I work on feeling into my own wings.

The wings I wear might be invisible and imaginary, but they have immense power. Like those of a dragonfly, they are beautiful and iridescent and allow me to fly in all directions, even when one breaks. My wings allow me to fly from dream to dream, navigating life's challenges with grace and ease.

What do you imagine your wings look like? How can you feel into your own beautiful, powerful wings?

It's all in your thoughts, in how you choose to frame your thinking. It's in how you use the power of imagination and consciousness. That is how humans endure harsh circumstances, cruel experiences, hatred, and racism. We allow our minds to go elsewhere, to dream, to take the higher road, to bypass the muck we find around us.

Your chakras are an internal reflection of the message of hope God gave to all of humanity eons ago. While it is certainly nice to see the vibrant visual reminder now and then, know that you are a living, breathing rainbow. Every day. Own that truth, that power, that beauty, that hope. As you meditate on your chakras, feel wrapped in infinite love. Shine your light, knowing deep in your body, mind, and soul that you were born for a reason. You are a miracle. You have purpose. It's time to speak and live out your truths. You can endure anything. You are extraordinary.

I have seen God's light in so many people and situations—in my daughters' eyes, in the way a five year old holds their friend's hand when they know their friend is too scared to talk in front of the class, in a much-needed hug, in the clouds, in the serene diamond-speckled landscape of a winter forest, in the way people speak up and demand change when innocent lives are being lost, in the way strangers come together to help a neighbor during their darkest hour, in the passionate voice of my pastor, in the way the tiniest of flowers grows through miniscule cracks in pavement, in the loving energy present during yoga class, in laughter and smiles, in good times and bad. God's light is always present, guiding us, illuminating us, and encouraging us to shine our own light.

As I am always pondering and wondering about all things related to spirit, I asked Roslyn McGrath, a healer and empowered light worker from Northern Michigan, to do an Akashic Records reading for me, in real time, right before the coronavirus became "real" in March. I am no expert on this topic, just seriously curious. Basically, The Akashic Records are a record of each soul's journey, in all times; past, present, and future. Think of it as a heavenly library or the universe's database. Akashic comes from the Sanskrit word "akasha," which means sky or space. Some in this field reference the Book of Life, mentioned in the Old Testament of the Bible. It was such an incredible experience. Roslyn was told that in my first incarnation I was one of the first angels and that I need to "feel into my wings." After that, I was like a hybrid creature— part angel, part human. Apparently, I've also reincarnated over 100,000 times, this being my last.

What? Is this for real? No wonder I feel so connected to the Divine and feel that my time on earth is almost through. I have no expectations to live up to. That's what she was told by my spirit guides or angels. There are no must dos that I must do. That's great. That Akashic Records reading gave me much to reflect on.

In my heart, I know I don't "have" to do anything to please anybody or please God. In reality, though, I still felt so full of passion to do so much, while at the same time giving thanks for the extended corona-time to work on my writing with *zero* obligations except for my family. That freedom went away when we went back to school in the fall of 2020. I felt the complete opposite. Like I was placed back on a running treadmill moving at top speed. Everything was hard. But again, that's another story.

Show Up

All I can do is continue to show up, spread my wings, meditate and focus on the good, do the work, live my purpose every single second, and simply do "the next right thing." (Again, thank you *Frozen* and *Frozen II* for all your life lessons.) Because I know that my time on earth is short, I want to share what I've learned so far with my girls so they can go on to take action and follow their dreams. I want *you* to follow your dreams and not waste another second of your precious time on earth.

Here's how I take action. I strive to listen for God's wisdom and direction and to feel that enduring love in every way. I do this in many forms—through constant prayer, reading scripture and other books full of wisdom, meditation and concentrating on the universal power within, listening to my own divine intuition, tuning out my mind and tuning into nature, writing, skiing, running, yoga, talking to friends, listening to children, dancing, painting, shamanic journeying, and through simply being present and grateful. In turn, I feel completely connected to God, the universe, the dreams in my heart, and how I'm meant to serve.

Showing up is not always easy. Life is full of distractions. Life is full of responsibilities and commitments. That's why we must make it a priority to take an inventory of what we value most and how we choose to spend our time. Showing up takes a lot of practice. Eventually, it gets easier. But as always, change is the only constant. Your ability or desire to show up will ebb and flow. If yours doesn't, great. You can go ahead and skip this section.

I'm only kidding. Everyone has different strengths. I'm sure that is partially why I was so attracted to Erich. His steady, calm, consistent energy balances my highly charged, change with the moon cycle emotions. I go through periods where waking up at 5:00 a.m. is the last thing I want to do. When I eventually refocus and get back on the train, I'm reminded why I cherish that morning alone time. I have simply retreated from an argument with Erich or a battle with my girls plenty of times because it was just easier than dealing with the potential of losing my shit and doing the hard work of staying calm and problem solving.

Making the effort to show up for yourself, your family, your community, and your planet is always worth it. Make little changes that feel natural to you, small goals to help you on your journey. Maybe that's reading an affirmation every morning while you're waiting for your coffee to brew, writing your pearl of the day every night before going to bed, setting your alarm five minutes earlier every day until you're waking up with enough time to do something for yourself, or sending a card to a different friend every day just because.

Then start setting bigger goals. Sign up and train for a race, organize a community service project, do a month-long meditation challenge—whatever pushes you a little bit outside your comfort zone is where you need to be. Reconnect with the dreams in your heart, follow your intuition and use it to steer you in the right direction, use your passions to spread joy and make a difference. Get some mantras in your head to repeat, or write them down and post them somewhere highly visible at home or at work to remind yourself of this important piece of your training plan. Eyes up. Rise up.

Be a Light

My ultimate dream is to be God's light. I wake up every single day with this purpose. I want to use my God-given gifts and talents to serve God by serving others. I want to be a light. I am constantly thinking about this and praying that what I'm doing is making a difference and lining up with this goal. This focus helps ground and center me, gives me purpose and hope, and provides answers and clarity to life's difficult questions.

Earlier, I told you about the many earthly dreams I have yet to accomplish. However, the dreams in my heart are really quite simple: 1) To be the best mom and role model I can and raise children who love God with all their heart, who grow up to be humble, kind, good, and faithful servants themselves, who also listen to the dreams of their hearts; 2) To inspire children (whoever I encounter in life, really, because I truly believe they are placed in my path for a reason) to know they are loved beyond measure, to look for the pearl in every day and in everyone, to simply live with joy and gratitude, and to believe they can do whatever they set their minds to.

One ultimate goal to rest my running shoes on is to be a good and faithful servant to the most extraordinary God. I can handle that. When I get old and gray, when I can no longer shuffle along on my skinny skis, I can still be a light to the One who loved me before I knew who I was. To the One who gave me my wings and gave me the courage to spread them wide and fly. I will remain true, and I will love forever.

I'll keep on being the best mom I can be and trying to inspire others until the day I die—and on into eternity. I hope and pray that while my spirit soars into the most beautiful of places, my legacy will live on and through my children, and grandchildren, and great-grandchildren, and on and on, just as my ancestors live on in me. The web of life woven together over time creates the most divine images. We can only imagine the ultimate design until we pass through heaven's pearly gates.

While we make the journey up the mountain, we are called to shine our light for others in any way possible. We are called to shine our own light as brightly as possible to add our own unique beauty to the world. We must stay true to ourselves. We must walk through periods of darkness with hopeful hearts. We must let others light the way when we can't see it for ourselves. We must honor all lights and all paths, as we are all simply walking each other home.

Though the waves may crash
And the wind doth blow
My soul remains untouched
I shall forever remain
Unaffected by chaos
My roots reach deep into Mother Earth
Drinking in truth
Absorbed in the rich soil of pure integrity
My limbs extend out
Stretching toward my final resting place
Happy to bend in the wind
and release what hinders my earthly growth
Though parts of me may break
Though people might try to cut me down

Trying to drown out my voice, my courage, my strength to stand strong
My spirit is forever flying
My essence lives on
In the rocks, in the water, in the air
While I remain rooted to the ground
I send forth my seeds of love, hope, honesty, service, determination, grit, light
The caged bird continues to sing
The willow continues to sway
The real me must carry on

Chandra Ziegler
October 27, 2020

Marquette Marathon

It was my constant positive, forward-thinking mindset, my stubborn personality, my dreamer mentality, my dragonfly wings, my sheer will and determination (along with the support of my amazing husband Erich) that brought me to the starting line of the Marquette Marathon in the beautiful Upper Peninsula of Michigan.

There I stood on a cool, dark morning, at the start line, which begins twentyish miles away from Marquette in Ishpeming with my BRF (best running friend), Kara Graci, to my right—who, by the way, ended up qualifying for the Boston Marathon. She'll write her own book someday with all her remarkable stories.

I was nervous, anxious, proud, hopeful, ready, not ready, all the feels. *Just shoot the damn start gun already! 26.2 miles of running will be nothing,* I thought as I reached up to rub my shoulders and felt the screws protruding under the thin layer of skin covering my collarbone.

BAM. The gun went off. Adrenaline pulsed through my veins. "I can't believe I'm doing this," I declared to Kara.

I felt pretty good for nine miles. It's amazing what that surge of adrenaline can do to your body and mind. It's powerful stuff. I tried not to think about the fact that the longest run I had done in the weeks leading up to this race was five miles. But then the negative self-talk crept in and made me seriously doubt myself from miles ten through sixteen. I was ready to quit.

I can't do this. I'm tired. You should be proud of yourself for making it this far. There's no way you can make it sixteen more miles! It's okay to DNF (did not finish) because you fucking broke your collarbone. And on and on.

Then Molly Smith, my cousin-in-law, and her fiancé Stephen gave me the loudest cheer at mile fourteen, even though I told her I probably wouldn't make it that far. At mile fifteen, I got a baby high-five from a stranger. And then an angel named Wayne swooped in at mile sixteen and asked me how I was doing. I told him my story and tried to hold back the tears. He stuck with me for two miles.

Wayne asked me how many marathons I'd done. "Four," I said. When I asked him the same question, he said, "Two-hundred-fifty-four." Was he for real? He must have been an angel. Maybe I was hallucinating.

In any case, Wayne gave me advice that carried me (slowly) to the finish.

At mile seventeen, Megan, Mary, Anne, and Cory, my girlfriends from Duluth, sent texts that boosted my spirits. At mile nineteen, Erich was there to walk with me. "I'll be at the finish, and I expect to see you there."

Okay. Somewhere along the bike path, the self-talk changed.

Just keep putting one foot in front of the other. Spread your wings. Expect miracles. I am a warrior.

A dragonfly flew with me around mile twenty-three. A deer leaped right in front of me at mile twenty-five. Then there was Kara, screaming at me and cheering me on after finishing her own race. She ran with me up Third Street in Marquette. That long uphill finish was just the jagged icing on top of a brutal cake.

I crossed the finish line with a primal scream like never before and fell to my knees. The nurses asked me if I was okay. I just wept. Hell, yes I was okay! I fucking finished. I had *finished* it.

Six weeks prior, I didn't even think I could be there. During the race, I didn't think I could finish. But I did, and I couldn't have been more proud. The journey getting there and the 26.2-mile story were painful.

The beauty of a marathon is that it requires every single person to be the absolute best version of themselves. The connections (and disconnections) between mind, body, and soul required to succeed are intense. When your body starts to fail, you have to let your mind take over and battle those negative thoughts. In the end, your spirit takes over and pushes you to the end, and you realize it was your powerful spirit plus the amazing energy of those around you that carried you from the beginning.

You know what got me to that finish line? You could call it stubborn determination or something else. I call it love. I finished because I love myself. I show up, and I don't give up. I dream, and then I take action. I did it for myself and nobody else. I wasn't trying to prove anything to anyone. I definitely

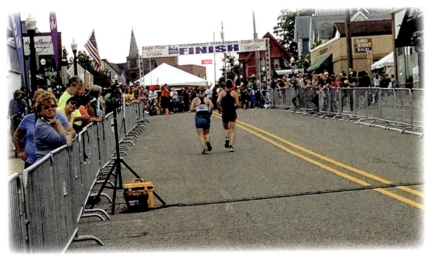

Finishing the Marquette Marathon just six weeks after breaking my collarbone. September 2018.

knew I wasn't going to qualify for the Boston Marathon. I also knew I might not finish. I knew it was going to be painful and ugly and fucking hard. But I made a promise to myself, and when you love yourself enough, you finish what you start.

Connecting

Here are other ways I connect with my third eye chakra and take action to get things done:

- I manifest them into reality. Yep.

- One of my spirituality classes was about manifestation. During an exercise, I visualized manifesting my dream of qualifying for the Boston Marathon. I had a clear image of finishing a marathon with the clock reading 3:28. It'll happen. Just watch.

- I've manifested so much already. But I'm never on my own. I know that.

- Through all the Energetically Simple Circle classes we discussed many topics, which allowed my spirit to grow and feel connected in many new ways. I gave myself time to tune in to my intuition. I believe all the knowledge, wisdom, love, and guidance I received from the amazing women from this circle provided me with support and inspiration. I discovered some pretty cool stuff that explained exactly why I live the way I live. I have a sense of urgency every day. I have so many things I want to accomplish, and I feel like I need to go after all of them at

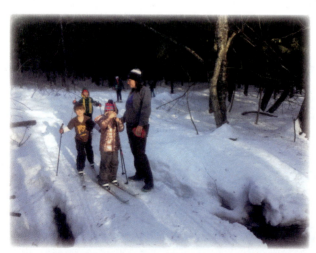

Kids skiing as part of Iron Endurance's after-school ski and snowshoe club.

the same time. I've always had this deep feeling that life is short. Now I know why. This is my last life on earth. Then it's off to the Universe to guide others on their journeys.

Leading a kids' yoga class.

- If I don't like something or I see a need, I don't point fingers, complain, or waste energy—I just create change.

- There's no track for the track team? Are you serious? Well, at least I tried to make that one happen. Someday.

- There's no yoga studio in town? I'll teach yoga. And still maybe someday I'll open my own studio (where we'll do yoga, I'll lead meditation classes, sell amazing books, be and build social justice warriors, spread light and love, and pure awesomeness).

- There's no group to get kids on trails? There's no bookstore? I'll fix that.

- I work really hard to follow Albert Einstein's advice: "Our task must be to free ourselves…by widening our circle of compassion to embrace all living creatures and the whole of nature and its beauty." It takes a lot of effort sometimes to focus on the positive and keep my vibrations rippling at the highest frequency. This is especially true when it comes to people who purposely harm others or harm the earth. We must speak out against this while at the same time embracing them. It could look like writing a letter to a representative and then saying a little prayer for their wellbeing. Always send love and light when doing the tough things.

- I also work hard to heed the advice of Mother Teresa: "We need to find God, and he cannot be found in noise and restlessness. God is the friend of silence. See how nature—trees, flowers, grass—grows in silence; see the stars, the moon, and the sun, how they move in silence…. We need silence to be able to touch souls." Amen.

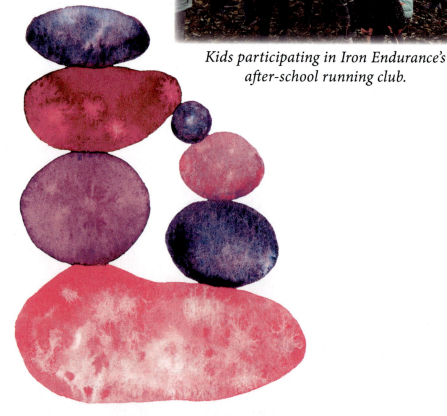

Kids participating in Iron Endurance's after-school running club.

"Intuition is the whisper of the soul."

— *J. Krishnamurt*

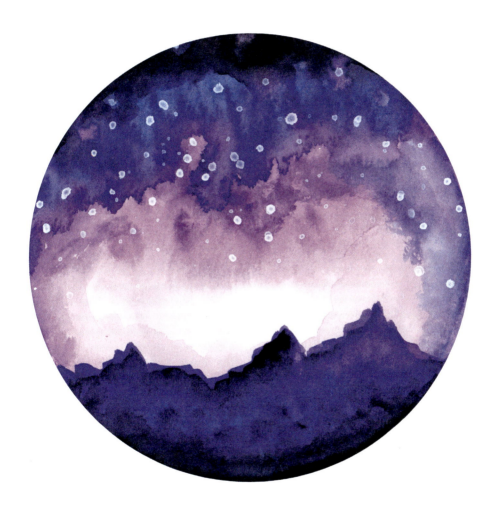

Chakra Guiding Questions

Third Eye Chakra

Close your eyes and draw your attention to the space between your eyebrows. This is your third eye chakra. The seat of your intuition. Take a deep breath in through your nose. Let it out slowly. Just listen and notice.

_____

_____

_____

What is your inner voice telling you? Listen. Don't judge. Just notice.

_____

_____

_____

Are you open to receiving Divine messages? If not, what small thing can you change to be more open?

_____

_____

_____

What messages have you received lately? These could be whispers during meditation, signs in nature, spirit animal messages, song lyrics that speak to your soul, numbers, a phone call, a knock at the door, the loss of a job, the deep desire to do something different, a recurring dream. Pay attention to your thoughts as you receive these Divine messages, and your path will be made clear.

_____

_____

_____

Chakra Training Tips

Third Eye Chakra

Visualization: As you inhale and exhale, picture an indigo ball of energy in your mind's eye. Breathe in and imagine it expanding all around your head. Breathe out and let go of all attachments. Continue breathing and notice your ability to dream, visualize, and connect with your intuition becoming stronger and stronger. Visualize your mind illuminating until you feel completely clear.

Positive Affirmations: I trust my inner wisdom and intuition. I am divinely guided. I see my path clearly. I pursue my dreams. I am healing in body, mind, and spirit.

Crystal Therapy: Lapis lazuli, amethyst, blue quartz, purple fluorite.

Nutrition: Blue-purple foods, caffeine, chocolate, spices.

Aromatherapy: Clary sage, cypress, frankincense, patchouli, rosemary, sandalwood, Douglas fir, copaiba.

Sound Therapy: Bells and chimes, chant *ksham* in the key of A.

Yoga Poses: Child pose, standing forward bend, seated forward bend, down dog.

Healing with Nature: Sit quietly in nature in the sunlight.

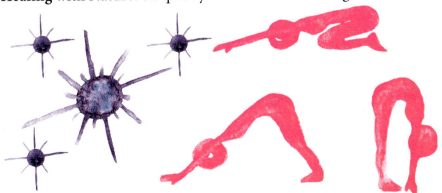

Be Extraordinary

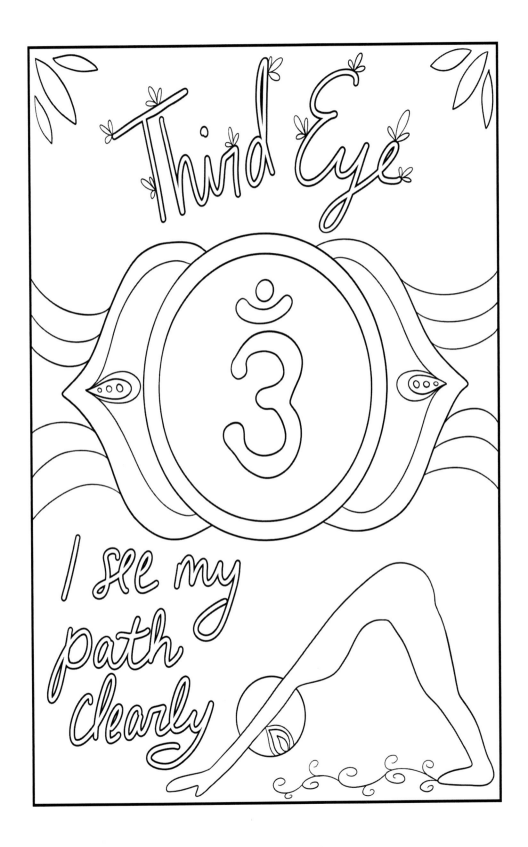

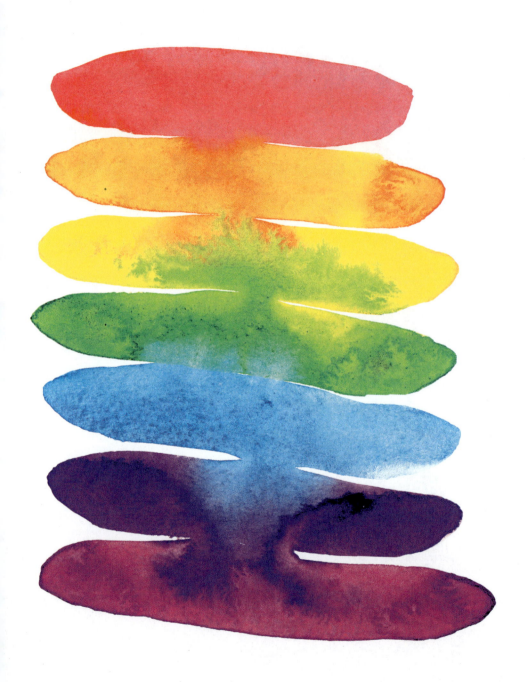

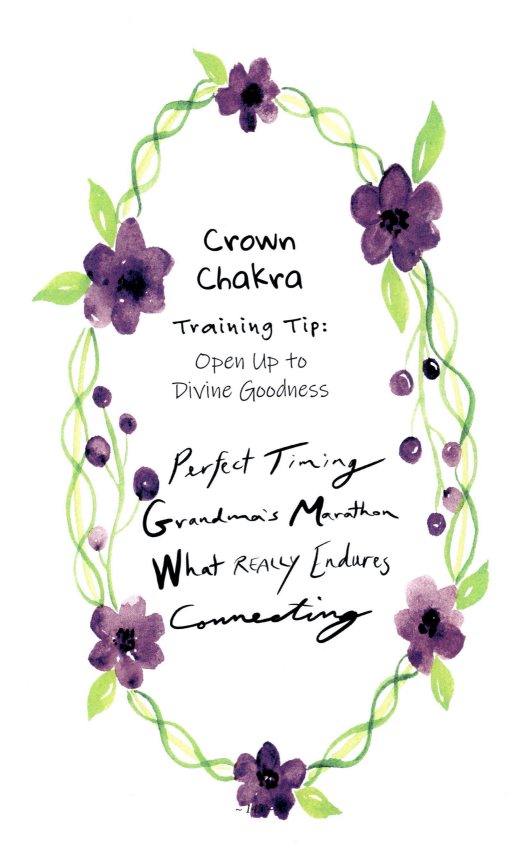

Crown Chakra

Training Tip:
Open Up to
Divine Goodness

Perfect Timing

Grandma's Marathon

What REALLY Endures

Connecting

You are filled with love
and light.

You are protected by love
and light.

You are called to shine
your light.

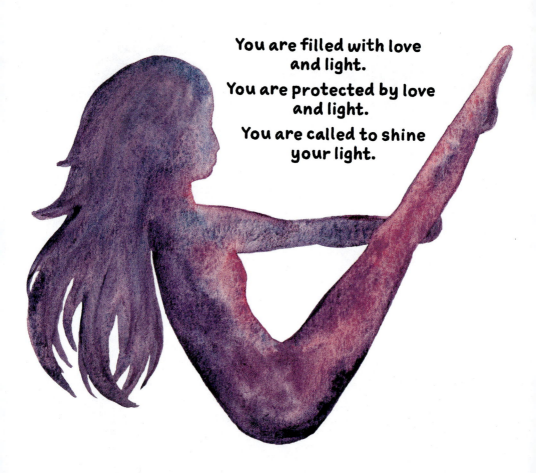

Perfect Timing

Knowing that each day is a true gift from above, it's with an eager heart and open mind that I attend church and soak in all the Divine goodness. Every time I attend my church, Grace Covenant in Iron River, Michigan, which I love dearly—the people, the praise, the incredible presence of spirit moving and at work—I am inspired. I am inspired to live more like Jesus, to live a purpose-driven life, and to love deeply.

On one particular Sunday, Covenant Point Director Erik Strom spoke about what really endures, what really matters. The message revolved around the following verse found in Isaiah 40:31: "Those who hope in the Lord will renew their strength. They will soar on wings like eagles; they will run and not grow weary, they will walk and not be faint."

Erik spoke so eloquently about the topic that he left me feeling great hope. His message also struck a very personal chord. I have endured a lot over more miles and races than I can count. Pain. Suffering. Frustration. Disappointment. Joy. Success. Freedom. Elation. I have learned more about myself while on a trail than anywhere else.

Since I was in middle school, and to this very day, every race I start begins with a prayer to God, giving thanks for my health, for getting me to the start line, and for the opportunity to serve. I view every race as an offering to God and an opportunity to be in harmony with the Holy Spirit. Leading up to those races are many solo training sessions. I have always used those miles as prayer in motion. I talk to God all the time on my runs, bike rides, and ski journeys. I also use that personal alone time to pray for others and our world.

I believe with all my heart and soul what the Psalmist wrote a long time ago, so I will always "Give thanks to the Lord for He is good. His love endures forever."

My first experience with trying to qualify for the Boston Marathon was on a horribly hot and humid day when the black caution flags were flying and thousands of people dropped out. I finished, but twenty-five minutes off of a BQ (Boston Qualifying) time. The second attempt didn't happen either (that was the broken clavicle race).

So as I sat in church listening to Erik's message, knowing I had less than two weeks until Grandma's Marathon...my third attempt at qualifying, I mentally took note of the impeccably perfect timing of the Scripture. I hope in the Lord. Hope is sometimes all I can fall back on. But knowing that gives me strength because I know when I start to grow weary on race day, I will pray even harder and be lifted up and soar on wings like eagles. I will run and be weary no more. God's great love will allow me to endure the 26.2 miles with a happy, happy heart.

Grandma's Marathon

All things in life come full circle. The Earth continues to spin, and we end up where we started. The moon travels around the Earth. Together, they make a full circle trip around the sun. We come from the spirit world, and when our time on this physical Earth is through, we once again return to that beautiful world of spirit. In the time between those bookends are multiple circles of various kinds. As a woman, there's the lovely monthly cycle. But there are as many different circles as there are humans inhabiting this planet. So it comes with no surprise that I'm ending this book back at the beginning—at yet another starting line. This time, where I grew up on the north shore of Lake Superior, at the start of the 2019 Grandma's Marathon.

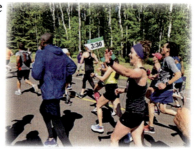

As with life, this marathon was more about the journey than the destination. The process of planning, training, and breathing through the tough stuff brought me great joy and peace. I was just happy to be healthy again and in (relatively) peak condition.

Waving to my support crew sometime before the halfway mark. Still smiling. June 2019.

You couldn't have asked for better weather for the race. A very different story from three years earlier. I toed the line wearing a headband with the verse from Isaiah that Erik had shared a few weeks prior. Not a coincidence. Just a mini-miracle. That verse became my mantra.

My mom and dad stayed with Kate and cheered from the house while the rest of the support crew, Erich, Greg, Rachel, Emma, and Hali, loaded into my parents' Subaru. Greg drove while my sister, who timed out precisely when I would be where along the 26.2-mile stretch from Two Harbors to Canal Park in downtown Duluth, expertly navigated the back roads to get to several spots in time to cheer me on.

They were adorned with rainbow unicorn horns and loudly rang their cowbells. Their yells of encouragement gave me the extra boost of energy I needed each time to keep pushing myself to the finish line. The second to last spot of their super-fan support team journey was on the slight downhill behind Fitgers. This was a reroute due to road construction. Typically, running downhill should come as a reprieve, but after twenty-three miles of pounding pavement at an eight-minute pace that about killed me. Not only was my body falling apart, but my mind was on some other plane. I didn't even see or hear them shouting my name and telling me how awesome I was doing. The pictures they captured of me at this moment truly summarize the struggle I was in.

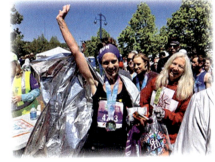

I stuck with the pacer until three miles to go. She slowly drifted away, and I fought to keep her in sight. I kept running as things became blurry. I became dizzy and nauseous. I heard my sister yelling with only a few hundred meters to go, "Every second counts!" And then I fought to get to the line in time. I finished in 3:34.19. That's a BQ, baby!

After crossing the finish line, I was a bit woozy. This angel of a volunteer stayed with me as I wobbled my way through the crowds to find my family, who captured this moment of pure joy. June 2019.

With only a forty-one-second buffer, I wasn't sure it would be good enough to race in Boston (they take the fastest first until each age group is filled). It was tough. But I couldn't do anything about it. Whatever happened, I was proud. I set a personal record by twenty minutes. I achieved my goal of running a Boston Qualifying time. I did it!

I waited three months to find out that my time was indeed not fast enough. There are too many fast people out there. Of course, I was bummed. But Boston will always be there, and I will train for it again. Someday, I will get my unicorn.

The extraordinary endurance needed to complete a marathon never ceases to amaze me. It's what brings me back to sign up for race after race. For the chance to give just a little extra. For the opportunity to be more than ordinary. To endure. To live. To light up the world.

What Really Endures

After the race was over, I began to think...maybe all the various interpretations of my dreams were accurate. Maybe I was the person getting in my own way. Maybe breaking my clavicle was the "external change" that needed to happen or at least the impetus for a bigger external change (aka coronavirus). Maybe I was still a little uncomfortable with the unknown direction I felt my spirit was leading me in after this major roadblock. I kept thinking, *So now what?* The truth is, I still can't quite make out the finish line in real life, so it is no wonder I can't finish the race in my dreams.

But here's the not-so-coincidental thing. After I finally got my BQ, I never had that dream again. So, I'm starting to believe that the journey to the finish line is becoming clearer by the day.

I will continue to dream, to write, to show up, to speak up, to teach, to listen, to learn, to live, to run. It's in my blood. It's in my heart.

As my feet hit the ground and pound, pound, pound away
to the beat of my heart
to the beat of the wind moving through the trees
to the beat of the music
I feel my purpose pulse through my veins
I feel connected to my ancestors who ran for survival
I feel connected to my creator and to family members who ran
this earth along with Jesus
I feel connected to the source of life alive within **all** of us
to the stardust that traverses the veins of all humankind
As my feet carry me forward
my mind unwinds
my heart expands
my hope is restored
I visualize the colorful threads of all my dreams reaching out into
infinity
I visualize all my dreams coming to fruition
I visualize the future in bright and brilliant colors
I run to become a better me
I run for peace
I run for those who can't
With every step of every run
I give thanks
I give thanks
I give thanks

Chandra Ziegler
October 25, 2020

My ability to keep going, to never give up, and to finish
what I start is a gift from above. I thank God for that gift, and
I continuously find great strength and peace in God's Word.
Romans 15:4-5 teaches us:

> For everything that was written in the past was written
> to teach us, so that through the endurance taught in
> the Scriptures and the encouragement they provide we
> might have hope. May the God who gives endurance

and encouragement give you the same attitude of mind toward each other that Christ Jesus had.

Let us learn from the past and learn from each other. Let us endure. Let us continue to encourage one another and above all *love* one another. I know it's not always easy. We will be confronted with many difficult situations. With all the news, all the hardships, all the expectations, all the stress, it can sometimes feel easier just to wallow and stay low or just live comfortably and not push any buttons. It might even seem unnatural or just plain impossible to live with joy and think positively. But if we change our attitude and choose to endure because we know it's good for us, we'll be okay. James 1:2-4 provides us with some hope:

> Consider it pure joy, my brothers and sisters, whenever you face trials of many kinds, because you know that the testing of your faith produces perseverance. Let perseverance finish its work so that you may be mature and complete, not lacking anything.

As does Romans 5:3-5:

> More than that, we rejoice in our sufferings, knowing that suffering produces endurance, and endurance produces character, and character produces hope, and hope does not put us to shame, because God's love has been poured into our hearts through the Holy Spirit who has been given to us.

The Bible sure has a lot to say about endurance. I take that as a huge comfort. In the end, here are some things that endure forever:

faith   *peace*

hope   *Love*

joy

I will continue to have faith in a force larger than all of us. A force capable of designing the most brilliant and beautiful creations. A force that allows us to learn from our own struggles, for it is in that struggle that we discover our strength and continue to strive. A force that gives me freedom to live as I choose and loves me unconditionally.

I will continue to hope for my family, my students, my friends, and the world and to dream big dreams for myself. I will continue to serve whoever or whatever is in my path, whether it's by teaching for another fifteen years, doing the dishes, raising our daughters, picking up garbage, weeding my garden beds, or going on a book tour. I believe hope and service to others will change the world.

I will continue to be peace and teach peace. If I pass you in the hall or on the street, know that I am silently sending you as much peaceful energy as I can possibly muster in the moment. I will let it radiate from the sacred space inside me and fill every corner of every heart in every room.

I will continue to love with a wide-open heart chakra. I will love deeply and passionately, and when I feel my heart getting too full or too heavy, I will use my own tips to bring balance and return to center, and hopefully after reading this, you can too.

I will continue to do what brings me joy and fill my days will smiles and laughter. I will radiate positivity as much as possible. I will keep running and skiing, painting and playing, looking at the clouds and looking for adventure, and appreciating all the little things.

And lastly, through my silent sports and my spirituality, I will forever continue to focus on love, no matter what. God's *love* is what really endures. That's what ultimately matters above all else. And when we love others, we will endure forever, for God is Love. And true love such as this requires the most extraordinary endurance known to humanity, for it is eternal. It is a "race" that never ends.

Love has extraordinary power, extraordinary healing, extraordinary everything. So, let's all go ahead and choke down an energy packet (or five) of *love* energy and carry on toward our ultimate finish lines. Amen?

Remember, life itself is a marathon. You are training your body, mind, and spirit for a lifelong pursuit of happiness and well-being. So take it easy, one step at a time; just breathe, and keep those chakras balanced in order to let your incredible rainbow light shine brightly.

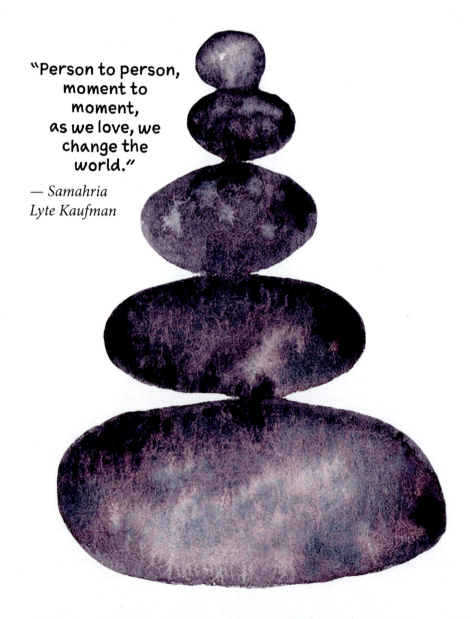

"Person to person, moment to moment, as we love, we change the world."

— *Samahria Lyte Kaufman*

Connecting

Here are other ways I connect with my crown chakra and open up to the divine goodness all around me—and what you can do as well.

- I imagine a thousand-petal lotus at the crown of my head opening to all the spiritual energy that vibrates throughout any space I enter.

- I understand that muddy waters nurture me and allow me to grow and bloom.

- I meditate often and pray throughout the day.

- I relish miraculous moments of blissful silence.

- I listen to OM meditations.

- I chant OM with my daughters on occasion.

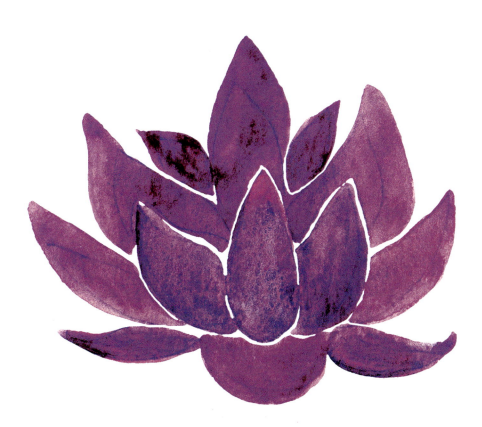

"You are a beloved of the Universe.

You are as beautiful as the sunrise and as ancient as the stars.

You are a spark of Divine love in human form.

Through you, goodness and light flow into this world.

Bless you."

— *Laurel Bleadon-Maffei*

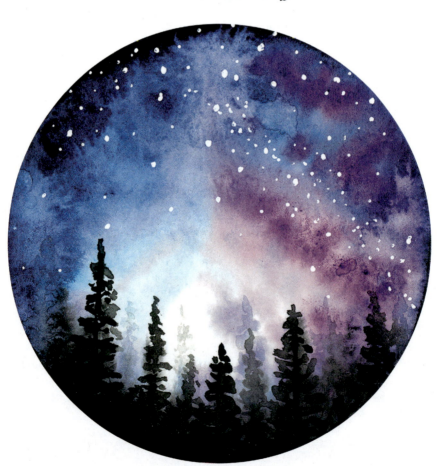

Chakra Guiding Questions

Crown Chakra

Close your eyes and focus on the top of your head, your crown chakra. This is your connection to the spirit world. Connect with all the Divine goodness radiating invisibly out, around, and within you. Check in. How does it feel? Where are you? Not feeling anything? Focus on your lower chakras for a while and try again later. You'll eventually feel light, happy, carefree, and full of love and peace. This is you, your true self, blissfully and effortlessly communing with God, the Universe, Love itself.

How does it feel to connect with the divine?

_____

_____

_____

How can you stay connected even during times of stress?

_____

_____

_____

How do you live a life filled with love?

_____

_____

_____

If you are feeling disbelief, fear, hate, distress, despair, what's one small step you can take to change those feelings to faith, hope, love, peace, and joy?

_____

_____

_____

How will you spread goodness and light upon the earth?

_____

_____

_____

NOTES:

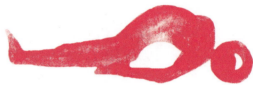

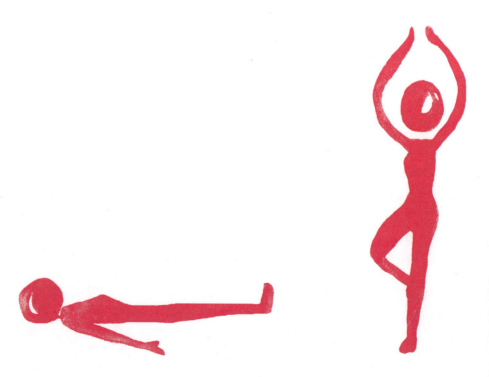

Chakra Training Tips

Crown Chakra

Visualization: As you inhale and exhale, picture a lotus flower, the ultimate purity of energy, inside the top of your head. Breathe in and imagine the lotus flower opening and enlarging your field of consciousness. Breathe out and imagine the energy spreading out into the universe. Feel a deep connection to the higher vibrational energies that fill you with love and light.

Positive Affirmations: I honor the spirit within me and all living things. I embrace the unity of all beings. I release all attachment. I invite sacred transformation.

Crystal Therapy: White calcite, white topaz, clear quartz, diamond.

Nutrition: Fasting and detoxification practices, no foods, toxin-free foods.

Aromatherapy: Sandalwood, frankincense, arborvitae, myrrh, rose.

Sound Therapy: Chant OM in the key of B, silence.

Yoga Poses: Headstand, tree pose, fish, savasana.

Healing with Nature: Go for a run, participate in any meditative or spiritual practice.

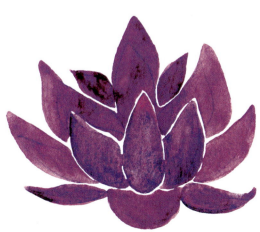

Be Extraordinary

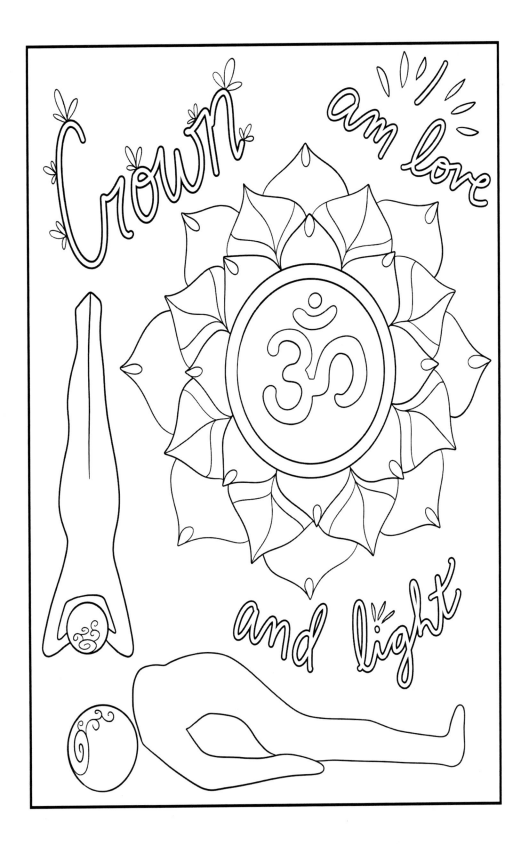

"The conclusion is always the same:
Love is the most powerful and still most
unknown energy of the world."

— *Pierre Teilhard de Chardin*

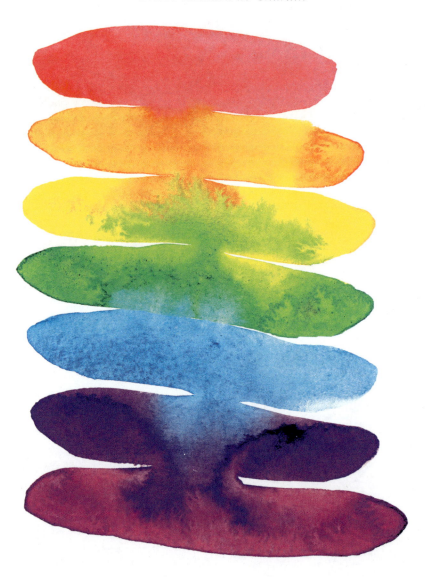

Rainbow Reflections

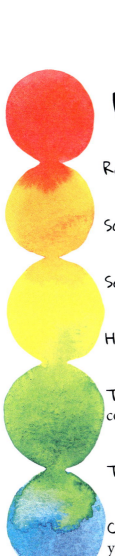

Root: Connect to the earth.

I am...

Sacral: Be creative.

I feel...

Solar Plexus: Stay strong.

I do...

Heart: Do whatever makes your heart happy.

I love...

Throat: Speak your truth…use your voice for the common good.

I speak...

Third Eye: Trust your intuition.

I see...

Crown: Slow down and take time to connect to your Higher Power, your source of divinity, to the extraordinary cosmos of light and love. Connect with family and friends and people in need, and show your love.

I understand...

Namaste?

Namaste!

My older brother Ben pulling my sister and I in the sled.

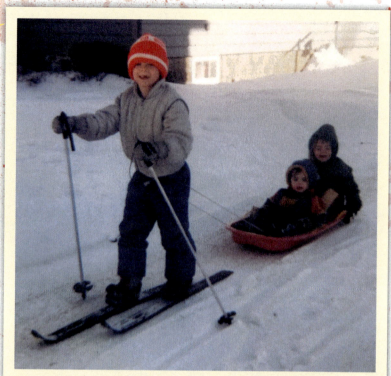

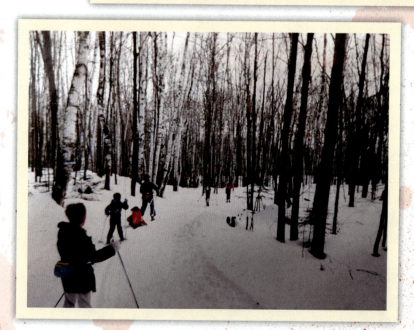

Out for a ski with family and friends. My mom is pulling one of us kids in their DIY kid carrier.

Here I am lined up for my very first ski race at age four with my dad giving direction and encouragement.

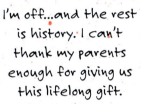

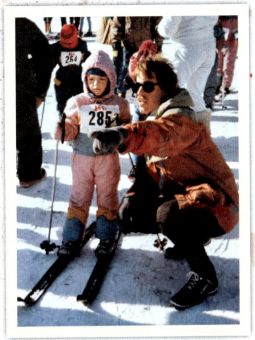

I'm off...and the rest is history. I can't thank my parents enough for giving us this lifelong gift.

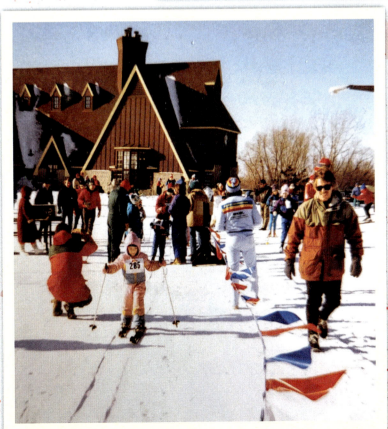

Lining up for a race. I'm bib 254. About 2nd or 3rd grade.

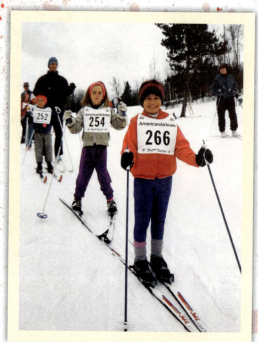

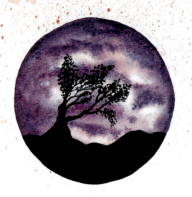

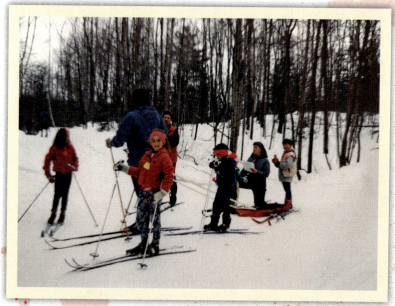

Another family ski outing. I'm front and center in my stylish flower pants and pink polar fleece jacket and pink headband.

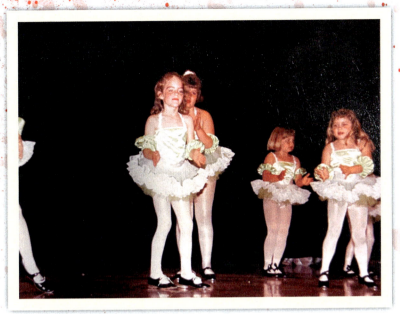

I took dance lessons from when I was 2 until I was about 10. I loved to dance, still do! Here I am front and center during a recital. I was probably in first grade.

Me, on the right, with my best friend Emily and her brother Grant during a talk show put on in her backyard.

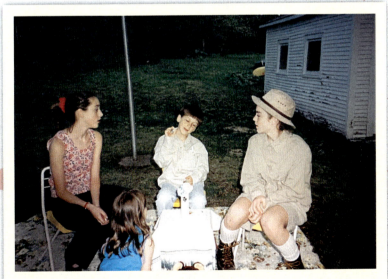

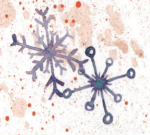

Flying to the finish line in Apple Valley, Minnesota as a 7th grader, 1996.

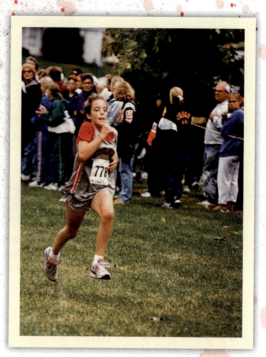

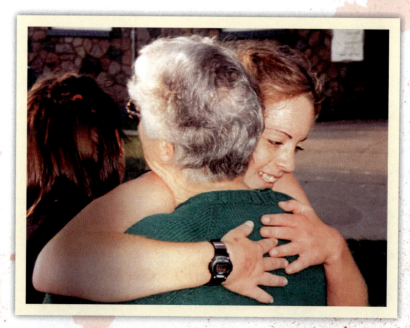

Hugging my grandma Jean after a race, sophomore year of high school.

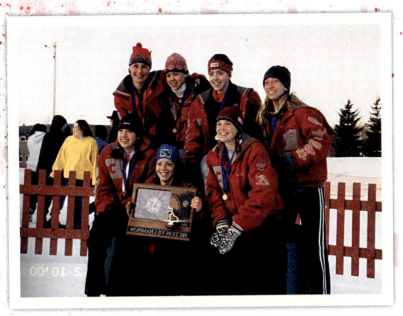

Section 7 Champions in nordic skiing! Go Greyhounds! I'm proudly holding the trophy, 2000.

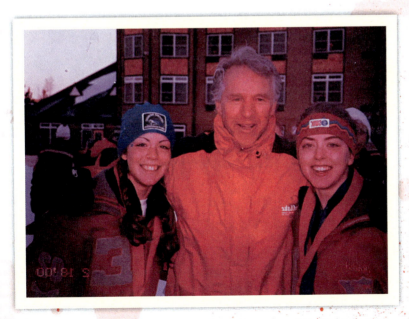

My sister Rachel, George Hovland, and I after a ski race at Giants Ridge in Minnesota, 2000.

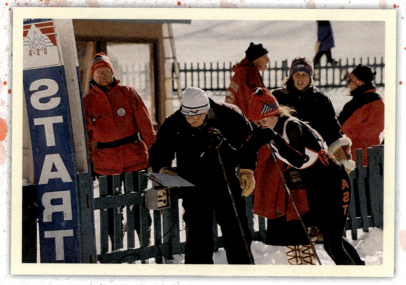

Focused and ready at the start of a race.
Giants Ridge, Minnesota, 2001.

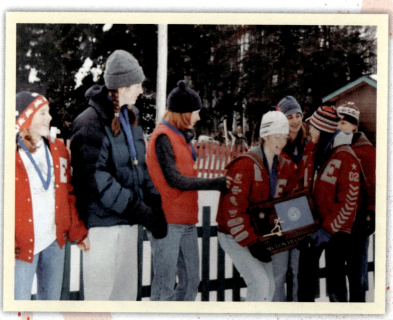

Senior year of high school with the honor of holding yet another
Section 7 Champion trophy for skiing with my teammates.
Giants Ridge, Minnesota, 2002.

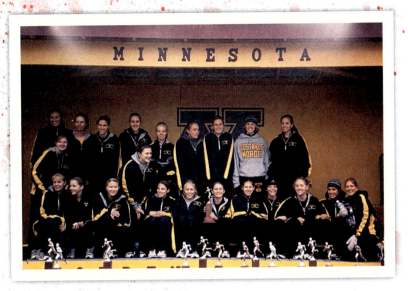

Gustavus Adolphus College cross country running team on the podium at the Roy Griak cross country meet in Minnesota, 2003. I'm in the front row, fourth from the right.

Finishing up a hard rollerski workout during college while visiting my grandma's house on break in Markesan, Wisconsin.

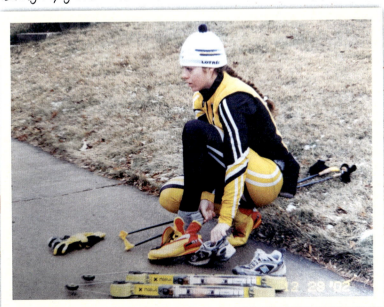

Ready to hammer up a hill at a cross country meet at St. Olaf College in Minnesota my senior year, fall 2005.

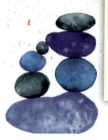

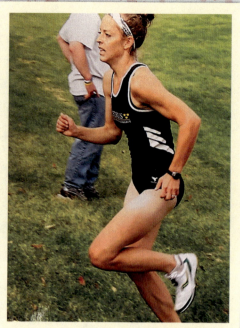

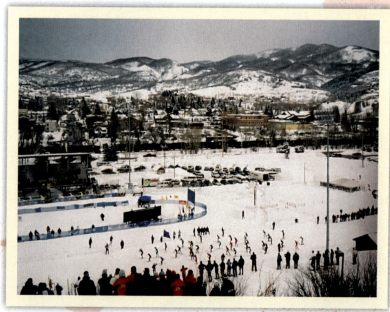

The start venue of the 5km skate race in Steamboat Springs, CO at NCAAs, 2006

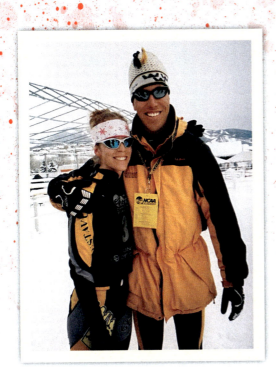

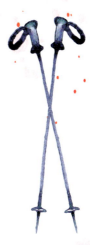

Me with my coach, Jed Friedrich, at the 2006 NCAA Nordic Skiing Championships

Me with my coach, Jed Friedrich at the 2006 Division I Nordic Skiing Championships in Steamboat Springs, CO.

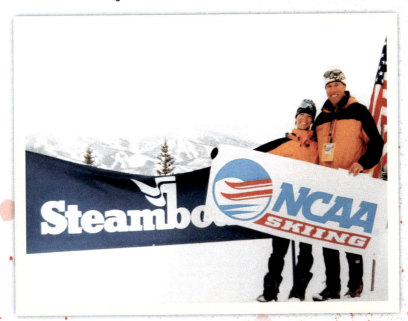

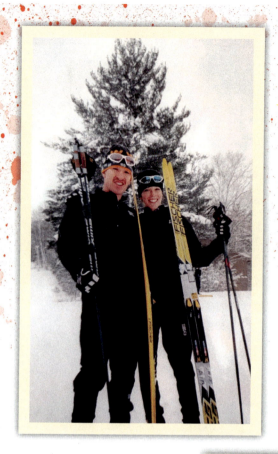

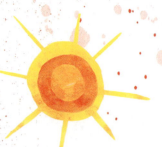

My husband Erich and I after one of many collegiate ski races.

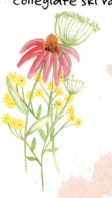

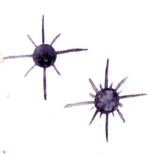

The best coach of all time, Dave Johnson, prepping me at the start of yet another race.

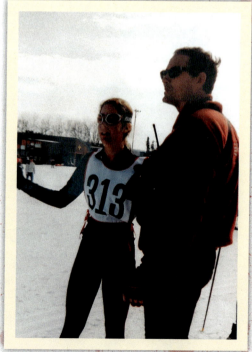

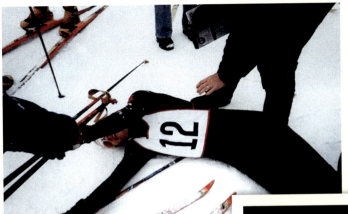

I gave my all in every race. They truly prepared me for life. You get out what you put in.

My mom enjoying the sights and sounds and stillness of the Boundary Waters on one of our many trips. I have a picture of myself in that same tree. Our love for wild spaces runs deep.

My mom and dad cheering me on in a college race during a blizzard with my grandparents cowbell from Switzerland. They went all in as a support crew!

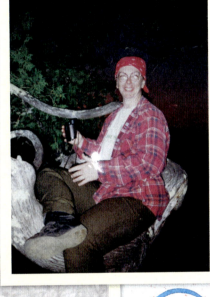

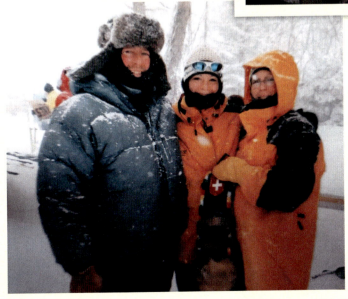

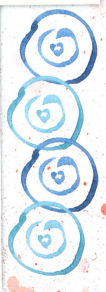

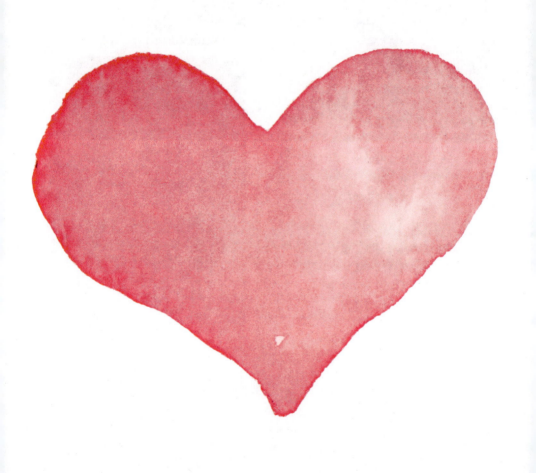

Acknowledgments

Thank you, dear reader, for coming along on this journey with me. I first want to take a moment to acknowledge you. You are amazing just by being you. You have so much to offer the world, and I wish you the best as you continue on your journey.

This book would not exist without the love and support of so many wonderful people.

To my husband, Erich, you are my rock. You are the home I always return to after spending time up in the clouds. Thank you for believing in all my crazy dreams, for pushing me out the door to run when I didn't feel like going, for being the best dad to our girls, for all your hard work, for your commitment to the well-being of all the students and staff you serve, and for your unwavering love.

To Emma, Hali, and Kate, I love you more than all the stars in the sky. Thank you for choosing me to be your mom. Thank you for your snuggles and providing me with so much inspiration. You make life so fun and keep me grounded in the present. You are my greatest joy and treasured gift. Thank you for letting me write just a little longer when you were hungry in the morning. Thank you for calling me out when necessary. Thank you for your unending love. I can't wait to watch how you grow and see where your wings take you.

To my parents, thank you for raising me so I learned to show deep reverence for our earth, for letting me be a kid, for buying me sketch books and running shoes as birthday presents, for not giving me everything I wanted, for always being there, and for your continued support. I love you.

To my in-laws, Bill and Joyce Ziegler, thank you for raising such an amazing son, for helping Erich and me with the girls, for all the Sunday night meals, and for your incredible love and support.

To Cheryle and Floyd Dropps, you might not be blood, but you are family. Thank you for always being there to help celebrate all the big milestones, for watching the girls when they were sick, for campfire stories, pontoon rides, and the best venison sausage around. I love you lots.

To all my teachers and coaches, many heartfelt thanks to you, for creating a strong foundation from which I could fly, for opening my eyes and mind, for believing in me and pushing me to be my best. You deserve more acknowledgment than these few lines can provide. You are all heroes. Keep doing your heroic work. It doesn't go unnoticed. You make more of a difference than you'll ever truly realize.

To the many mentors in my life, to my sister Rachel Bristow, to all my Gustavus professors, but especially Jill Potts, to my cooperating teacher during student teaching, the remarkable Karen Ferrington, to Kay (my first teaching partner who died tragically the year after we met; I know you're flying free and happy), to Verl Hudson and Nancy Hronkin-Force, both such wonderful, kind, strong role models during my early years of teaching who spread love and light and left others feeling better and who always sparkled bright, to Suzanne Standerford for helping foster my love for writing and teaching others to love writing, thank you all for your support, inspiration, ideas, and guidance.

To my past and present colleagues, your dedication to education is an inspiration! A special shout out to my current partner in crime, the incredible Lauri Patterson, who celebrated her thirtieth year teaching amid a global pandemic! We've collaborated together, cried together, complained together, and crushed teaching COVID-style together. You are amazing and I am blessed to work with you every day. Thank you, for everything.

To my Energetically Simple Circle and Yoga Tribe, thank you for your love and encouragement. Your positive energy lifted me and gave me the much-needed wind beneath my wings to get this book back in the air. Keep grounding yourself and working into those wings. I can't wait to get back to burning sage with all y'all.

To Kara Graci, my BRF, though we didn't grow up together, didn't go to school together, and have never lived in the same town, I consider you one of my closest friends. From UPWP to DID to Boston chasing training days, to surprise birthday burrito runs, and much more, I've come to value our long-distance relationship. You are raw and real and simply remarkable, my friend. I know you can do anything you set your mind to. Someday, we'll run another race together. Until then, keep training for life.

To my soul sisters, Megan, Mary, Anne, and Cory, to Emily, to Jen, to Lindsey, thank you for being the best friends a girl could ask for. You've been there for me through it all. Thank you for making me laugh, for cheering me on, for your lengthy text messages, for your surprise care package during my recovery. I can't wait to see what we're all up to when we're eighty-eight. I love you so much.

To all my family and friends, thank you for making me who I am, for making me laugh, for cheering me on, and for your enduring love and friendship. I love you all so much. You're all rock stars!

To my anonymous biker friend, thank you for getting me out on some of the sweetest single track, for building my confidence and ease with rocky terrain, for encouraging me to keep going after the crash. I appreciate having a wise biker buddy and look forward to many more tales from the trails.

To our Chariot, you have been a trusty and reliable baby hauler. How do I express my gratitude? Over the years, you have brought much sanity to my life. Thank you for never letting me make excuses and allowing me to get out the door with my little ones. Together, we've probably logged over 5,000 miles. You've made me stronger, tougher, and more resilient. As Kate will be turning four this year, our time together is nearly through. So to you, dear Chariot, I say thanks, and enjoy your retirement (or next family).

To Keneu and Fischer, two of the most faithful training partners and untrained therapy dogs on the planet! Keneu, you were our first baby and have witnessed much joy and sorrow and every emotion in between for the past thirteen years. Fischer, you are your own breed and we love you even more than the Fischer skis you're named after. BLBL is our unwritten family motto: Be Like a Black Lab.

To Cynthia Drake and Charli Mills, thank you for providing the time and space in your inspiring home that allowed me to bring my little sprout of a book to light. You were the first people who saw a tiny piece of this book. That writing retreat gave me the push I needed to continue. Thank you for your kind words and love and sharing your light.

To Amanda Rasner, I am so grateful that you reached out to me to read my book. I trusted you completely. Your suggestions and support were exactly what I needed. I knew we (DJ included) were meant to be friends before we even met, and I can't wait to see how our life journeys continue to entwine.

To Melanie Bess, you've always been a breath of fresh air. At board meetings, yoga classes, family photo shoots, or other gatherings, you were always calm and confident. Your energy is so delightfully positive. I adore you as a person and a friend. I'm in love with your artwork, and I couldn't think of any other person to partner with in creating this book. Thank you for dreaming right along with me in bringing this book to life. Cheers to rose-colored glasses and to all the dreams in our hearts!

To Tyler Tichelaar and Larry Alexander of Superior Book Productions, for your superior editing and design knowledge and services. I appreciate all the time and energy you poured into this project. Thank you for helping bring my dream to reality.

To all the people I have met along the way, I know our paths crossed for a reason. Thank you. Keep shining your light.

Resources

Crystal Therapy

This is the "newest" alternative medicine I have been reading about and practicing a bit. Basically, crystals come from the earth and hold various properties that help facilitate healing. They act as a conduit to aid in absorbing positive energy and ward off negative energy. They are closely linked with the chakra centers and the areas of the physical body those chakras are connected to. I am not a scientist nor an expert. What I do have is an open mind. That is essential with every mode of alternative healing. The mind is our superpower.

For a more personal testimonial of the natural healing power of crystals, I reached out to my friend Gina Onderak, a certified Reiki II and shamanic practitioner. Her words speak such truth, and they make me realize I have been tapping into this earthly energy since I was a kid. I, too, have such a connection to rocks. They are everywhere in my house, in the car, in my husband's boat. As Gina describes, they are like friends that cheer me up. I am especially connected to rocks that come from the shores of Lake Superior. They make me feel grounded and connected.

As Gina describes, the funny thing about "crystals" is that in my life they came along long before books and mentors or resources on the internet about spirituality and energetic healing. It started on the big lake, Superior, and during a very difficult time in my life. Walking along the beach was a great source of comfort. Allowing all the accumulated stress to flow through me. The crashing waves pulling it away. My favorite beaches were covered in water-washed stones. As I walked, I would stop to pick up and examine those that called me. Like others who love the beach, my car, pockets, and home were filled with the treasures I found while walking.

They lined the windowsills in my apartment, filled the cup holders of my car, and my favorites were in the bottom of my purse.

My beach combing turned into a full-blown passion. Geology clubs, rock swaps, tailing piles of mines long forgotten was how I spent any free time. Extra money was used to buy the tools of the trade and travel to new collection points. The funny thing was that the joy of collecting wasn't the only benefit.

One specific day I remember clearly. My husband and young son were out collecting with our local geology group. We had permission to collect in a closed mine. There was specifically a space where they had dumped truckloads of crushed hematite to be processed. Piles of hematite that had been pulled from the earth—tons and tons. Some of it was what was considered specular hematite, there was peacock ore, and lots of pockets of quartz crystals. I have never felt so grounded. Each piece I picked up was calling to come home with me. To this day, hematite is one of my greatest allies.

Fast forward a decade and I found myself exploring alternative healing. At first, I was put off by the large volume crystal-wearing, high-vibration, everything is love and light members of the healing community. I also knew many of the "crystals" being offered for sale as "healing tools" were glass, plastic, chemically altered, or dyed.

As energetic beings, we interact with the world around us. As spiritual beings, the world around us wants to support us on our journey. This process happens in multiple ways. Just like teachers, each stone has strengths to share with everyone and the ability to form relationships with an individual to support them in specific ways.

There are stones that have amazing healing properties, some for protection or clearing energy; others invoke a feeling of peace and gratitude.

Choose a stone you are drawn to. How does it feel? Think about what task you would like it to help with.

Quartz in all its forms is an amazing place to start. Amethyst, Rose, Smokey or Clear, it carries a very clear high vibrational energy, intuition, and healing. Tiger's Eye for strength, power. Hematite is amazing for calming anxiety and grounding. Tourmaline to connect to your roots and remember where you came from.

If you are starting to work with stones, allow your intuition to guide you. The most powerful tool may be the one a child finds out in the yard. What calls to you as an individual? Like a friend, appreciate the qualities you find when working with individual crystals or stones. If you do purchase something...and you find it doesn't have the qualities you were looking for, pass it along. You may give someone exactly what they were looking for.

Sitting with a stone in meditation, keeping it in your pocket or close to your heart, placing it in a space where you will often see it and be reminded of the task you asked it to help with are all ways you can simply incorporate gemstones into your daily life.

Nutrition

The Rainbow Diet and Chakra Foods for Optimal Health by Dr. Deeana Minich are two excellent resources for more in-depth information about the healing powers of food. Dr. Minich also created a simple road map of sorts called "The Seven Systems of Health" that includes foods, physiological issues, and more.

Some of my favorite ways of incorporating the rainbow in my diet is through smoothies, soups, salads, and hummus. From a simple base, you can get creative and add just about anything to make it more colorful and bursting with flavor and nutrition.

Sound Therapy

Sound has been used as a tool for healing by many different cultures for thousands of years. There's no denying the fact that music or sound can affect our emotions and attitudes. Science backs this up. According to Mind Body Green, sound helps to facilitate shifts in our brainwave state by using entrainment. Entrainment synchronizes our fluctuating brainwaves by providing a stable frequency the brainwave can attune to. By using rhythm and frequency, we can entrain our brainwaves, and it then becomes possible to down-shift our normal beta state (normal waking consciousness) to alpha (relaxed consciousness), and even reach theta (meditative state) and delta (sleep; where internal healing can occur).

By focusing on the pure sounds from tools like drums, singing bowls, tuning forks, or by holding notes at a certain frequency, you can mold your mind. This is a quick and easy way to help you slow down and bring about a more relaxed state of mind. From this state comes peace, calm, and the ability to live with pure clarity and realize our thoughts, problems, or whatever we're currently living through is just temporary.

Yogapedia explains that chanting certain one-syllable sounds specific to each chakra can be done to ease energetic blockages or imbalances. Focus on the inner vibration while you chant to bring about greater self-awareness. The chakras and their corresponding syllable to chant are as follows:

- *Muladhara*, or root chakra - *lam*
- Svadhisthana, or sacral chakra - *vam*
- Manipura, or solar plexus chakra - *ram*
- Anahata, or heart chakra - *yam*
- Vishuddhi, or throat chakra - *ham/hum*
- Ajna, or third eye chakra - *om*
- Sahasrara, or crown chakra - silent om

Listening to Native American drumming or the chanting of Om for five minutes can have a significant positive effect on your emotions and well-being. When you allow yourself to be mindful in the moment, focused only on the sounds and the present, you will feel immediate shifts as your body adapts physically to your more peaceful state of mind.

Aromatherapy

Smell (specifically for the training tips in this book, essential oils) has also been used as a tool for healing by many different cultures for thousands of years. There's also no denying the fact that smell can affect our emotions and even our memories. Science also backs this up. According to Dr. Brent A. Bauer, MD at the Mayo Clinic, aromatherapy works by "stimulating smell receptors in the nose, which then send messages through the nervous system to the limbic system—the part of the brain that controls emotions."

Plenty of testimonials and case studies are all over the place about how well they work. I, for one, can personally attest to the positive benefits of using essential oils in my own life, with my children, and in my classroom.

doTERRA is my go to for the best essential oils on the market. doTERRA sources and provides the purest, highest-grade essential oils. Before I became a conscious consumer, I would buy essential oils from department stores that were on sale for five dollars, thinking I was getting a bargain. Well, sometimes you get what you pay for, folks. I also got a pretty bad rash. No longer.

"Through industry-leading, responsible sourcing practices, doTERRA maintains the highest levels of quality, purity, and sustainability in partnerships with local growers around the globe through Co-Impact Sourcing®. The doTERRA Healing Hands Foundation®, a registered 501(c)(3) nonprofit organization, offers resources and tools to sourcing communities and charitable organizations to raise self-reliance, increase access to healthcare, promote education, advance sanitation, and fight against human trafficking. Through the life-enhancing benefits of essential oils, doTERRA is changing the world one drop, one person, one community at a time."

Interested in learning more? Check out my website: https://www.doterra.com/US/en/site/chandraziegler.

Yoga

What can I say about yoga that hasn't already been said? Yoga and mindfulness have been around for thousands of years.

According to Yogabasics, yoga's history has many places of obscurity and uncertainty due to its oral transmission of sacred texts and the secretive nature of its teachings. The early writings on yoga were transcribed on fragile palm leaves that were easily damaged, destroyed, or lost. The development of yoga can be traced back more than 5,000 years, but some researchers think yoga may be up to 10,000 years old. The beginnings of yoga were developed by the Indus-Sarasvati civilization in Northern India more than 5,000 years ago.

Yoga has spread far and wide as people from all walks of life have discovered its benefits.

I have read many books and articles on yoga and mindfulness.

I have participated in many different types of yoga classes.

I have taught yoga for years in my small town.

I have been practicing even longer.

My interest and knowledge continue to grow and evolve. Currently, I am participating in a program called Breathe For Change.

Breathe For Change is a movement enhancing the health and well-being of educators, students, and entire communities. Their mission is to Change the World, One Teacher at a Time.

They offer the world's only 200-hour Wellness, SEL, and Yoga Teacher training for educators and community leaders inspired to use wellness as a vehicle for healing and social change.

Breathe For Change's visionary curriculum is as grounded in truth as it is revolutionary. The program empowers educators to transform the system from the inside out, equipping us to courageously show up as our whole and brilliant selves, no matter what external pressures we face.

It's an amazing community! I am inspired every day. The passionate, huge-hearted, wellness-champion, social-justice warrior in me feels deeply at peace, overjoyed, and incredibly inspired by the journey I'm on. If you'd like to learn more, check out breatheforchange.com.

The most important thing to remember when doing yoga is to listen to your body. Don't overstretch, overextend, or overdo it. Just take it easy. Work on building up your stamina and flexibility over time. If you have any underlying conditions, consult with your doctor for more specific recommendations. Have fun with it, and allow it to transform you from within!

Chakras

One stroll through a bookstore will tell you people are very interested in personal growth. That gives me hope for our world. On my latest visit, the entryway of the store was flanked by a beautiful display of books about chakras, mindfulness, yoga, and the like. Inside, there were shelves upon shelves of books related to mind, body, spirit, and well-being. I was inspired. It's impossible to list my favorite resources here. I encourage you to browse your local bookstore and find one that speaks to you. Keep an open mind, and allow yourself to evolve!

Art Therapy

Although not mentioned in every training tip section, there is real value to be found in letting yourself get creative, so it's worth mentioning here. It's why we incorporated a coloring page with each chakra! We hope you enjoyed the time to color and unwind.

Whether through dancing, creating music, singing, painting, drawing, knitting, tying flies, etc., any art-form that requires your full attention is considered art therapy. It is a powerful modality of healing that allows people of all ages to express themselves. Participating in the arts roots you to the present, lowers your stress and anxiety, improves self-awareness and self-confidence, strengthens relationships, helps children regulate behaviors, and improves social skills. Although there is plenty of data backing up these statements, I don't need any studies to prove these things to me. I've felt the benefits for thirty-six years of my own life. I've witnessed the transformative nature of the arts as an educator for the past fifteen years. I've seen it all play out in front of me as a mother of three girls.

If you love the illustrations in this book as much as I do, you can find more of Melanie's work and support her at TheSwimmingOwl.com.

About the Author

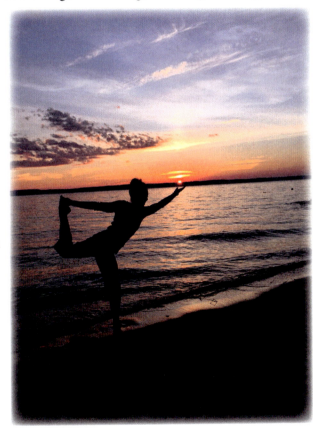

*C*handra Ziegler is a proud public school teacher, free-spirited dreamer, and the author of *Extraordinary Endurance*. Part memoir, part self-help, part journal, *Extraordinary Endurance* will inspire you and fill you with ideas on how to tap into your inner strength, live your best life, and achieve all your goals, both big and small. Chandra has been an endurance sport fanatic for more than twenty-five years and has completed thirty marathons. When not teaching, momming, running, writing, or studying to become a certified Social Emotional Learning Facilitator and Yoga Instructor, she can be found playing in the outdoors in the Upper Peninsula of Michigan with her husband, three daughters, and two black labs. To learn more about Chandra and her other endeavors, visit her at www.DreamStar Dragonfly.com.

About the Illustrator

Melanie Bess-Haight is a multi-passionate artist, creating in every available moment she can find. As a new mom, this typically means she is painting by the light of the moon. She has been doodling and creating since her toddler years, and that passion turned into a creative career that has spanned from photographing weddings to teaching art classes and now illustrating books. Her illustrations are typically inspired by nature with a touch of fantastical whimsy and heaps of color. She resides in the Upper Peninsula of Michigan along with her husband and daughter.

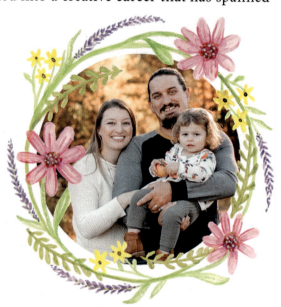

You can find Melanie's illustrations on art prints, coloring books, home decor items, tech accessories, apparel, and more. To learn more about Melanie or shop more of her artwork, visit her website www.TheSwimmingOwl.com.

Made in the USA
Columbia, SC
13 December 2021